A bet on Natural Endocrinology

Dr. Mario Vega Carbó
Endocrinologist

First Edition, July 2019

Copyright © 2019 Mario Vega
All rights reserved.

*To my daughters, Liuba and Rocio and my sons, Fidel
and Mario
To my parents, Lucia and Nicolas
To my wife, a Dr. Ethel Vado Osuna
To my partners, patients and their relatives
To God in nature, the best source of health*

CONTENTS

Introduction 7
Topic I Diabetes 9
Chapter 1 Definition 10
Chapter 2 Most frequent causes 12
Chapther 3 Most common symptoms 15
Chapter 4 Associated diseases 17
Chapter 5 Consequences, prevention and natural advices 19
Chapter 6 Treatments 25
Chapter 7 Physical activity and metabolic control 30
Chapter 8 Dietary measures 35
Chapter 9 Vitamins and minerals 42
Chapter 10 Medicinal plants 44
Chapter 11 Endorsed productos for diabetic people 47
Chapter 12 Alternative therapies for managing diabetes 50
Topic II Obesity 54
Chapter 1 Concept 55
Chapter 2 Most frequent causes 57
Chapter 3 Most common symptoms 60
Chapter 4 Associated diseases 62
Chapter 5 Consequences 64
Chapter 6 Treatments 66
Chapter 7 Physical activity 71
Chapter 8 Dietary measures 75
Chapter 9 Vitamins and minerals 82
Chapter 10 Medicinal plants 87
Chapter 11 Natural supplements 89
Chapter 12 Alternative therapies 92
Topic III Thyroid gland diseases 97

Chapter 1 Concept 98
Chapter 2 Most frequent causes 100
Chapter 3 Most frequent symtoms 102
Chapter 4 Associated diseases 105
Chapter 5 Consequences 107
Chapter 6 Treatments 110
Chapter 7 Physical activity 113
Chapter 8 Dietary measures 115
Chapter 9 Vitamins and minerals 124
Chapter 10 Medicinal plants 127
Chapter 11 Natural supplements 130
Chapter 12 Alternative therapies 132
Topic IV Polycistic Ovary Syndrome 134
Chapter 1 Concept 135
Chapter 2 Most frequent causes 137
Chapter 3 Most common symtomps 139
Chapter 4 Associated diseases 141
Chapter 5 Consequences 142
Chapter 6 Treatment 144
Chapter 7 Physical activity 147
Chapter 8 Dietary measures 149
Chapter 9 Vitamins and minerals 156
Chapter 10 Medicinal plants 159
Chapter 11 Natural supplements 161
Chapter 12 Alternative therapies 162
Topic V Menopuase e Andropause 164
Chapther 1 Concept 165
Chapter 2 Most frequent causes 167

Chapter 3 Most common symtoms 169
Chapter 4 Associated diseases 170
Chapter 5 Consequences 171
Chapter 6 Treatments 173
Chapter 7 Physical activity 177
Chapter 8 Dietary measures 180
Chapter 9 Vitamins and minerals 185
Chapter 10 Medicinal plants 188
Chapter 11 Natural supplements 191
Chapter 12 Alternative therapies 192
References organized by topics and chapters 195
The author 214

Introduction

The purpose of this book is to create awareness about the nature; it has all the nutrients that we need for a healthy diet, to prevent diseases, to relieve their symptoms and to battle against the effects of those that bring us to here: endocrine diseases.

It is not intended to replace the medical treatment, but open new options and possibilities to be encouraged, and having more options to choose.

We will do a trip to know the causes and consequences of five endocrine diseases which are taking control of our society and we will get prepared to struggle with them by using traditional therapies, but also natural measures, such as changes in lifestyle, diet, exercise, and resources that we can find in the plants, so as to be part of the treatment of these diseases.

We start with Diabetes. This is a clinical condition that has turn in to an epidemic nowadays. We will know which are the diagnostic criteria, its types and classification, alarming symptoms, and also the treatment, explaining the effect of drugs, the importance of a healthy lifestyle and which plants are beneficial to patients with diabetes.

Then we will continue with a topic strongly related to diabetes, which is Obesity. Nowadays, obesity is considered as a serious illness, a silent enemy that can lead to a lot of diseases and consequences. We will talk about types of obesity according to the accumulation of fatty tissue, consequences for health, and measures for non-pharmacological treatments, drugs that can be used and advised natural remedies.

As a third chapter we presented the Thyroid Gland and its diseases, which happen because of alterations in its functions. The thyroid gland produces hormones which are very important to boost metabolic processes in our cells; when this production is higher (hyperthyroidism) our lower (hypothyroidism) than the normal, it comes with lots of symptoms that affects all the systems in our organism. We will learn about causes, consequences, and alternatives to traditional medical therapies such as treatment with medicinal plants.

Chapter four is about one of the most prevalent diseases among women with infertility, this is Polycystic Ovary Syndrome (POC). Its prevalence is around 12% in women in reproductive age. We will explain the concept of this pathology, its symptoms, causes, and what conventional treatments are, and also natural measures that can be helpful to its management.

The last topic, it's a journey to prepare us to manage a difficult period of life, with several physical and psychological changes; this is the Menopause in women, and Andropause in men. We will talk about the reasons why these changes happen, its physiology according to age, symptoms, and also we will guide you to know therapies that can be adopted to overcome this period in life.

As you travel through the pages of this book, you will get more aware of everything that is in your hands to improve your lifestyle day by day, as soon as you wake up until you go to bed in the night. Since this moment, your life can change to be better; you just have to let the alchemy takes place. You are the wizard.

The author
Dr. Mario Vega Carbó

Topic I

Diabetes

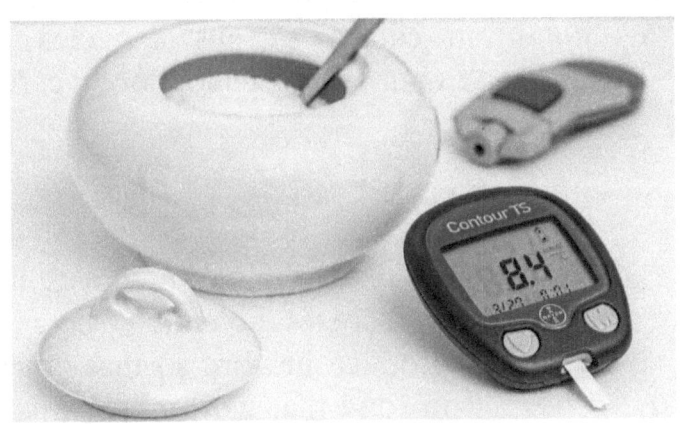

Chapter 1

Definition

Scientific definition: Diabetes is a chronic disease that occurs when the pancreas stops producing enough insulin to regulate the level of blood sugar. Also, when the pancreas produces insulin normally, but the body is not able to use it effectively, diabetes can be acquired. When this disease is not controlled, a condition known as hyperglycemia occurs in the body, it means that there is a level of blood sugar higher than normal. As time runs, this condition causes serious damages to the body's organs, also in our systems and blood vessels.

Pathophysiological classification:

Type 1 Diabetes: this type is also known as insulin-dependent diabetes or diabetes juvenile. Occurs when the pancreas cannot produce insulin, so that glucose in our body, presented in food that we eat, remains in the bloodstream, not being able to get in the cells, where it is necessary for its functions. These high levels of glucose in blood start causing a lot of consequences in the body which affects health. This diabetes doesn't have a way to be prevented.

Type 2 Diabetes: It is known as non- insulin – dependent or diabetes of adulthood. Type 2 occurs when the pancreas produces insulin but our organism is not able to use it because there is failure to transport glucose into the cells. In consequence, there are high levels of sugar in the bloodstream, which is harmful to health. When this type of diabetes starts cannot be noticed, in fact, a lot of people suffer from it for years, until finally there is a serious consequence that makes them notice there is something wrong, for example, eye diseases, heart diseases and others. Because of it, our organism is programmed to regenerate, when the liver and the fatty cells don't use insulin normally, pancreas starts producing more insulin to beat this resistance. However, there is a moment when the pancreas stops this effort, so insulin production decreases and the disease becomes aggravated.

Diabetes in pregnancy: This is a condition which is characterized by the presence of hyperglycemia, i.e., high levels of sugar in blood during the pregnancy. It happens because during this period there are lots of changes in the endocrine system which can lead to develop hyperglycemia. This represents a risk in pregnancy and the consequences can be labor problems, and higher risk to baby develop endocrine diseases, such as type 2 diabetes in the future.

Other types of diabetes: In this category are included those types of diabetes that are caused by a pathophysiology different from the previous one explained, generally the causes are as a result of another illness. For example, diabetes caused by steroids drugs, and diabetes cause by cystic fibrosis.

Chapter 2

Most frequent causes

Type 1 Diabetes

Today we just know very well the causes of type 1 diabetes which is autoimmunity. The scientists are researching about genetic aspects, as it is known that a person gets born with a genetic susceptibility, which could be activated for a viral infection, and in consequences, the immune system starts a reaction against the own pancreas cells, destroying those that produces insulin. In summary, the causes of this diabetes are mainly two:

- **Genetics**
- **Environmental risk**

Type 2 Diabetes

This type of diabetes is related strongly to lifestyle. Unhealthy habits such as sedentary lifestyle and unhealthy diet are at the top of the list of risk factors. This is because there is a proved connection between obesity an insulin resistance that leads to type 2 diabetes. Abdominal fatty tissue causes insulin resistance, but it is also a signal of disease. Another risk factor is genetic. The most vulnerable groups to suffer from this disease are Latin people, African American, North American, and people from pacific islands. In summary, the causes of this type of diabetes are:

- **Lifestyle**
- **Genetic**
- **Ethnicity and geographic location**

Diabetes in pregnancy

What happens in diabetes in pregnancy is caused by three main factors. First, genetic has an important influence, along with unhealthy lifestyle such as unhealthy diet and being sedentary. On the other hand, there are lots of hormonal changes during pregnancy so, all these factors interact together and lead to diabetes. One explanation talks about the actions of placental hormones act against the function of insulin. Also, gaining a lot of weight during pregnancy is another risk factor. In summary, causes for diabetes in pregnancy are:

- **Genetic**
- **Lifestyle**
- **Hormones**

Other types of Diabetes

Drugs

Other causes of diabetes are some drugs that can cause hyperglycemia and onset diabetes in a person that has vulnerability to this disease. Some of these drugs are: opioid analgesics, steroids, rheumatologic medications, some antibiotics, immunosuppressant and antineoplasics, hormones and bronchodilators.

Chapter 3

Most common symptoms

Our organism is very wise and instinctive; talking by symptoms it is expressing those troubles that aren't so evident. So that, when we see one or several of the following signals, we could be suffering from a silent diabetes and don't even know it.

Polyuria: it is too urinate in large volume. We shouldn't confuse it with urinate several times but small volume (polaquiuria).

Polydipsia: it is the excessive increase in thirst, which comes with an urgency to drink water. It makes the person drinks a lot of water our other types of liquid.

Polyphagy: it occurs when there is a feeling of hunger out of control, which makes the person to eat lot and many times during the day.

Weight loss: weight loss happens without any factor causing it, although the person is eating more, and there is no change in lifestyle or habits, without diet or exercise.

Other suspicious symptoms

Itching: itching of the skin without reason.

Fatigue: for no obvious reason, we feel tired and find hard to breathe when doing little physical effort.

Blurred vision: in this case we have to rule out sight tiredness, and pay attention if this symptom is occasional our continuous. It suggests diabetes when is constant in many circumstances.

Wounds that not heal: if you have wounds that take long time to heal or get infected frequently, you should look for diabetes.

Numbness and feeling of "ants" in arms and legs: when we feel this things and movement impairment constantly, it can be a signal of diabetes.

Chapter 4

Associated diseases

When, for lack of knowledge of negligence, we don't treat our diabetes, lots of consequences happen in the body that lead to diseases. Some of them are:

Candidiasis vaginal: it is a vaginal infection caused by fungi, which manifests by intense itching in the vaginal and vulvar area. Other symptoms that appear are rash, redness and pain as well as watery or thick vaginal secretions.

Balanitis: this is the inflammation and irritation of the glan or foreskin in men, and the clitoris in women. In this case appears redness, painful urination, purple and red sores in the area, and secretions from the urethra.

Urinary infections: it occurs when bacteria enter into the urethra and settle in the bladder. This infection can affect the urethra, bladder, ureters, or kidneys. Generally when bacteria get into the urinary system they are expelled and destroyed by the immune system. However, diabetes reduces the function of immune system making or organism weaker against bacteria and other microorganism, so infections can occur.

Skin infections: we have to pay attention on frequent skin diseases such as infections, because this can be an alarm signal of diabetes. If we have constantly boils, styes, abscesses… it could be because of diabetes.

Oral and dental diseases: when glucose is higher than normal in blood, the organism becomes more susceptible to suffer from oral and dental diseases, such as periodontitis, which can lead to lose teeth. There is a general deterioration on oral health. So that, it is very important to pay attention to these problems, and go to the dentist every six months, especially if we have diabetes.

Chapter 5

Consequences, prevention and natural advices for managing

When diabetes occurs, it comes with several consequences which are harmful to health. Fortunately, we can prevent them before they appear, and control them once they are established. These consequences can be the following diseases:

Peripheral neuropathy

The nerves that are out of the brain, which starts in the spinal cord, are the peripheral nerves which transmit sensitive information to the brain and carry commands to the organs and muscles. These are serious affected because of pathophysiology of diabetes, especially in arms and legs. In consequence, the patient has numbness and loss of sensation in feet and hands. Also, the patient feels tired and weak, with fatigue.

Preventive measures

- **Control the diseases that can cause it, such as:** diabetes, arthritis, alcoholism, Lyme's disease,

VIH, liver and kidney diseases, and troubles in the function of thyroid gland.
- **Avoid the contact with toxins**
- **Avoid repetitive movements**
- **Do exercise**
- **Consume vitamin B**
- **Consume lots of fruits and vegetables**

Natural advices to control it:

- **Consume walnuts**
- **Consume fish oil**
- **Take some sunbathing during 15' daily, as it increases the levels of vitamin D**
- **Consume wheat, herbs, and natural juices**
- **Consume chili peppers**

Sexual dysfunction

Sexual dysfunction is a condition when men lose erectile function and women lose sexual desire. To get this diagnose it is necessary have a persistent condition, without being related to psychological factors. The cause is the damage that suffers the peripheral nerves.

Preventive measures

- **Stop smoking**

- **Lose weight**
- **Sleep at least 7 hours per day**
- **Avoid stress**
- **Increase wellness**
- **Have a healthy diet**
- **Do exercise**

Natural advices to control it

- **Acupuncture**
- **Kegel exercises**
- **Consume ginseng**
- **Consume arginine**
- **Consume Ginkgo biloba**

Chronic kidney disease

We talk about chronic kidney disease when the damage on kidney physiology and function is serious, progressive and irreversible. In this case, the disease has started many years before the onset of symptoms, generally the person don't know it. To detect any damage on kidney function we can do some studies and tests such as glomerular filtration rate, blood urea and creatinine, urine test and blood pressure test.

Preventive measures

- **Control glucose level in blood**

- Do exercise, at least 30' per day, three days a week
- Don't smoke
- Reduce alcohol consume
- Control weight
- Control blood pressure
- Reduce the intake of fat food
- Reduce the intake of salt.

Natural advices to control it:

- Consume food rich in potassium and minerals
- Consume onion soup
- Drink infusions of bearberry, dandelion, horsetail and mauve.

Ischemic heart disease

It occurs when the wall of coronary arteries is damaged by a condition known as atherosclerosis, which leads to less irrigation to heart. Generally, at the beginning there aren't few symptoms, but it can cause anginas and heart attacks.

Preventive measures

- Avoid sedentary lifestyle

- **Don't smoke**
- **Have a healthy diet**
- **Reduce stress**

Natural advices to control it:

- **Consume nuts**
- **Consume onion**
- **Drink hawthorn infusions**
- **Consume avocados and plantains**
- **Consume honey**
- **Drink infusion of garlic and white vinegar with honey**
- **Drink mistletoe infusion**

Diabetic foot

Diabetic foot is a complication caused by loss sensation (peripheral neuropathy) and damaged blood vessels, it courses with loss sensation in feet which causes that if the person has a wound, it won't be noticed, and can advanced until sores and ulcers, which get infected and can lead to an amputation. Even a small wound can be the cause of a serious problem.

Preventive measures

- **Check feet everyday**
- **Wash feet daily**
- **Hydrate feet with creams**

- Be extremely careful when removing callosity
- Use shoes comfortable
- Avoid extreme temperatures
- Use socks

Natural advices to control it:

- Apply aloe Vera with essential oil of tea tree
- Take bath with sea salt
- Drink ginkgo biloba infusions
- Drink calendula infusion
- Apply coconut oil with vitamin E

Chapter 6

Treatments

Treatment for diabetes is based in a combination of non-pharmacological measures and drugs, which are progressive measures that are going to be implemented in each patient according to their individuality and differences.

The first step in treatment is always based in non-pharmacological measures; these are changes in lifestyle mainly. To reach weight loss, especially in patients with diabetes type 2 and obesity, it is necessary to keep a diet with low calories, planed according to the needs of each patient. The goal is losing 5% of the weight per year and keeps this weigh stable.

Also diet has to be combined with moderate to high intensity aerobic exercise, for 30' during at least three days per week. These routines need to be adapted to the person; they can be walking, jogging, or other types of exercise, always thinking in the comorbidities that the patient has.

When metabolic alteration in diabetes can be control just with these measures, medications are needed.

Medications

Medications are indicated in case of diabetes type 2. In this type of diabetes the main alteration is a resistance of the body tissues to the action of insulin, although the pancreas continues to produce insulin, but al lower levels than normal. For this reason, the drugs have two functions: (1) increase the production of insulin by the pancreas, and (2) improve the sensitivity of tissues to the action of insulin. There is a wide range of drugs that can be classified according to the way they act in the body as follow:

- **Biguanide:** the most known in Metformin. It works by improving the sensitivity of tissues to the action of insulin and is the first choice for patients with diabetes type 2. It is taken two or three times per day.
- **Dipeptidylpeptidase IV inhibitors:** in this group we find Sitagliptin, Vildagliptin and Saxagliptin. They act by blocking the action of an enzyme called Dipeptidyldipeptidase IV. This enzyme is a protein that is responsible for eliminating substances produced by the intestine, called incretins, which have the function of stimulating insulin production when food in ingested. They are taken orally.
- **Incretinomimetics:** in this group we have Exenatide and Liraglutide. These are medications that are injected. Their function is similar to the

effects that have the substances called "incretins"; it is to stimulate insulin production.
- **Thiazolidinediones:** such as Pioglitazone. It is a medication that is taken orally and its function is to improve the action of insulin in tissues, mainly acting on fatty tissue. In addition, they decrease the production of glucose by the liver. Among its adverse effects it has been related to weight gain and heart problems.
- **Meglitinides**: These medications are stimulants of insulin secretion by the pancreas and they are taken orally. As adverse effects they can cause hypoglycemia, i.e., lower levels of sugar in blood. Examples are Repaglinide and Nateglinide.
- **Sulfonylureas:** they are one of the most commonly used for the treatment of type 2 diabetes, alone or in combination with Metformin. These are stimulants of insulin secretion, and they're usually taken orally once a day. The main adverse effect is hypoglycemia. In this group we found such as: Glibenclamide, Glicazide, and Glimepiride.

Hormonal Therapy: Insulin

The therapy with insulin is given to patients with type 1 diabetes, pregnant women with type 1 or 2 diabetes, or diabetes in pregnancy, and also in patients with type 2 diabetes advanced. In cases of type 1 diabetes and type 2 diabetes advanced, the pancreas is not producing insulin, so that, the hormone needs to be replaced.

The insulin is injected, intravenously or subcutaneously. There are available some synthetic human insulin analogs and other types such as Insulin NPH, which are classified by the time they act in the body. These injections need to follow a very rigorous scheme, related to the periods of food and need to be controlled by determining capillary insulin with glucometer before eat. Nowadays there are also available scheduled insulin pumps to help patients in the administration of insulin automatically.

Risks and benefits

The side effects of the medication are varied and depend on the type of drug. In general, the most common are hypoglycemia, nausea, diarrhea, vomiting, weight gain and decreased sodium in the blood. Talking about benefits, these medications have the function of increasing insulin production, helping the body use it correctly and making the liver produce less glucose.

Surgeries

- **Diabetic food surgery**
- **Pancreas transplant**
- **Surgery to treat obesity**

Indications, risks and benefits

Diabetic foot surgery is recommended when facing a foot at risk, which implies that an amputation may be needed if the wound persists and cannot be cured by drugs. The risk of this surgery is related to the difficulty for healing presented by the diabetic patient, while the benefits are restoring the health and preventing more infections.

In the case of pancreas transplant we find other risks to consider. The first is the seriousness of the intervention. In fact, 20% of the transplanted people die within the first year after the operation. On the other hand, the side effects of immunosuppressive medications that must be taken to prevent the body from rejecting the new organ are more dangerous than diabetes itself.

Surgery for the treatment of obesity is considered because many patients with type 2 diabetes are obese. Surgery is indicated in cases where the BMI is greater than 40 kg / m^2 and also when the value is between 30-39 kg / m^2 and the patient has not been able to lose weight by conventional measures (diet and exercise), and when other serious associated diseases are presented, such as high blood pressure.

Chapter 7

Physical activity and metabolic control

Physical activity influence on metabolic control

Doing a strict and regular metabolic control is what will take us away from the complications derived from diabetes.
Exercising has a highly positive impact on people with type 1 and type 2 diabetes. Besides of getting all the benefits that physical exercise brings, diabetic people will acquire the following advantages:

- Improves the levels of glucose in blood
- Increases the sensitivity to insulin

At the metabolic level, what happens when you exercise is directly related to diabetes, it is the mobilization of glycogen deposits in the liver and muscles. In addition, the muscles begin to absorb glucose, so they take it out of the blood. Finally, physical exercise, especially aerobic, triggers the burning of lipids, which improves the action of insulin in the tissues, leading to lower blood glucose.

Kids and adolescents with type 1 diabetes are able to perform any type of physical activity, they can even practice competitive sports, but they must always have adequate metabolic control. To perform physical activity safely, it is necessary to adapt the medications and diet.

Associated diseases and consequences

The most common associated diseases to diabetes are those affecting small blood vessels:

Retinopathy: occurs because high blood sugar levels damage the blood vessels of the retina. In consequence, the vessels swell and lose fluid or new abnormal vessels are formed. Over time, all these changes can lead to loss of vision.

Nephropathy: is the chronic kidney disease, which results in poor filtration of blood by the kidneys and dangerous accumulation of waste and electrolytes in the body.
Neuropathy: peripheral nerves are weakened, which leads to numbness and loss of mobility of body parts.
As well as **cardiovascular ones (angina, heart attack)**, which are associated with metabolic control and disease evolution.

Combined exercise routines: resistance, cardio, flexibility and elasticity

There are some exercises especially recommended for people with diabetes. Although, when practicing physical activity, its four pillars must be considered, it is necessary to emphasize that the most beneficial for metabolic control to take place in people with this disease is aerobic exercise.

So as to get the benefits derived from physical exercise, this should consist of sessions for at least thirty minutes of uninterrupted exercise, and that take place at least three times per week.

Routines can be chosen according to time and energy available. To have the desired effect, aerobic exercise must last between twenty-five and forty-five minutes.

Aerobic/ Cardio exercise

- Cycling
- Skating
- Elliptical
- Quick walk
- Swimming
- Dance
- Running

Resistance

When talking about resistance, we refer to the use of weights to generate an increment in muscle mass. We must remember that the more volume in the muscle, the more glucose will be absorbed. The repetitions of the resistance exercises range between ten and thirty per series, and at least three sets must be performed. The muscles which need to work are:

- ABS
- Back muscles
- Arms
- Legs

Flexibility

There are routines for reach the widest range of movements in joints. These bring benefits for body position and movement. The most recommended are:

- Yoga
- Pilates
- Ballet

Elasticity

People with diabetes suffer from premature cell degeneration, so it is common for them to have joint wear, muscle tears and tendon injuries. To avoid this, exercises should end with a routine for muscle elasticity. Here the arms, legs and spine will be worked. With this we help muscle to receive the necessary nutrients and release the accumulated lactic acid in the resistance session and we can avoid feeling pain; each stretching exercise must last at least twenty seconds and be repeated twice.

Chapter 8

Dietary measures

Carbohydrate counting

Carbohydrate counting is a technique focused on controlling the blood glucose level through menu planning, knowing nutrient that raises glucose levels. However, if we want it to be effective, it is not as simple as adding the carbohydrates present in food, because two factors that reduce the effect of this nutrient must be taken into account: physical exercise and the medication.

On average, we can start from the basis that 52 carbohydrates are needed per meal. As an example, a breakfast with this amount of carbohydrates could be formed by:

- 1 fresh fruit
- ½ cup of oatmeal
- ½ cup of unsweetened yogurt without sugar
- 1 sweet cookie

Diet according to glycemic index and glycemic load

The **glycemic index** tells us about the speed at which a food is able to raise blood glucose. It is necessary to divide foods between those with low, medium and high glycemic index. The value of 100 is attributed to glucose. Therefore, those foods that are less than 55 have a low index; between 55 and 70 have intermediate and those above 70 have high index.

The **glycemic load** evaluates the speed at which glucose reaches the blood. In this case the carbohydrates contained in the food are evaluated. For example, if the food has a high glycemic index, but contains few carbohydrates, its glycemic load is low. You can't talk about glycemic index without taking into account glycemic load, and vice versa. Foods above 20 are considered high glycemic load, as they will make glucose reach the blood faster. Those under 10 are of low glycemic load

High glycemic index foods: white rice, watermelon, processed cereals, instant oatmeal, potatoes.
Medium glycemic index foods: brown rice, pita bread, rye bread, raisins.
Low glycemic foods: barley, quinoa, nuts, legumes, milk, yogurt

High glycemic load foods: pasta, sugar cereals and raisins
Medium glycemic load foods: bread, boiled potatoes, honey
Low glycemic load foods: pineapple, cereals with fiber, lentils, kiwifruit

Tag reading

Before buying any product it is good to read carefully its tag. The factors to take into account are the following:

- **Serving size:** the values that we read in the tag are per serving, not for the entire package. It is very important not to get confused and believe that we will eat only 52 calories if we consume the whole package, since we can be talking about that amount of calories for three cookies, for example.
- **Calories:** it is very important to consume fewer calories than the body is currently burning through physical activity to lose weight.
- **Carbohydrates:** include sugars, fiber and complex carbohydrates. Every carbohydrate raises blood sugar, so it is necessary to take into account the total grams, not just those of sugar.
- **Fiber:** it is advisable to eat an average of 25 grams per day in women and 38 grams in the case of men.
- **Alcohols and sugars:** they have fewer calories than carbohydrates and starch. You need to be careful because they can be present in a food whose label says "sugar free", which does not exempt it from carbohydrates or calories.
- **Total fats**: includes the count of bad and good fats for the body. Mono and polyunsaturated fats

reduce bad cholesterol and protect the cardiovascular system.
- **Saturated fats:** increase bad cholesterol and the risk of coronary heart disease.
- **Trans fats:** increase bad cholesterol and the risk of coronary heart disease.
- **Cholesterol:** the less it has, the healthier the food is. Ideally, say 0%
- **Sodium:** does not affect blood glucose, but the amount allowed to ingest daily is 2,300 mg.
- **List of ingredients:** they are listed in decreasing form. Thus, the first mentioned will be the one that is present to a greater extent.
- **Daily percentage values (%DV):** it is found at the right of the label we will find these values. It tells us the amount of each nutrient that each portion of the food contributes per day based on a 2,000-calorie diet.
- **Total Carbohydrates:** this is a value that has been included in tags currently. This is the amount of carbohydrates after subtracting sugar alcohols and grams of fiber. It is not a value accepted by food and diabetes organizations because it is not accurate.

Food recommended

People with diabetes get benefits from food rich in calcium, fiber, potassium, vitamins A, C, E, and magnesium. The following are recommended foods for them:

- Citrus
- Sweet potato
- Green vegetables
- Berries
- Natural beans
- Fish with Omega 3
- Whole grains (germ and bran)
- Tomato
- Walnuts
- Skim milk
- Skim yogurt

Most recommended recipes and quantities

The best diabetic dishes are: grilled, boiled, steamed and baked. It is better if you don't cook it too much, since this favors a greater absorption of carbohydrates. The best way to make a food dish for diabetics is:

- ½ dish of green vegetables (spinach, chard, carrots)
- ¼ dish of proteins (meat, tuna)
- ¼ dish whole grains or starchy foods (rice)
- Dessert: 1 fruit or 1 dairy product

It is good to eat the same quantity of carbohydrates daily.

Examples of menus

Breakfast

- 1 glass of milk
- ½ cup of oats
- 1 fruit

Lunch

- 1 cup of vegetables
- 1 portion of salad
- 1 fruit or dairy product

Snack

- 2 slices of bread
- 1 glass of de natural juice

Dinner

- 1 boiled potato
- 200 g of spinach
- 5 spoons of rice

Attractive and healthy culinary recipes

Hot or cold steamed salad:

- 2 carrots
- 1 zucchini shell
- 1 eggplant shell
- ½ onion

Cut the onion into julienne or brunoise, sautéed in a tablespoon of altoleic oil. Cut carrots into thin slices are added. Cover and let sweat. Add the rest of the ingredients seasoned to taste and then cover and allow completing cooking. It can be eaten cold to hot.

Baked stuffed tomatoes

- 4 tomatoes
- 4 potatoes
- 1 can of tuna
- 1 onion

Put the onion in a tablespoon of altoleic oil. Boil the potatoes and mash them. Peel and cut the tomatoes. Mix the mashed potatoes with the tuna and onion. Fill the tomatoes and cook 20 minutes in the oven 180 °C.

Chapter 9

Vitamins and minerals

All vitamins and minerals are beneficial for people with diabetes, but we will focus on those that not only nourish, but also reduce the level of blood glucose, either because they break down fat, because they reduce the presence of blood glucose, because they provide energy that otherwise we would have to get from carbohydrates or because they stimulate insulin production:

- **Vitamin B**
- **Vitamin C**
- **Vitamin D**
- **Vitamin E**
- **Magnesium**
- **Zinc**

Food rich in vitamins and minerals

- Nuts
- Cereals
- Cheese
- Oysters
- Citrus
- Wheat derivatives
- Raw seeds

- Beer yeast
- Mushrooms
- Milk
- Vegetables
- Locust
- Fish
- Green vegetables
- Tea
- Cocoa milk
- Celery
- Broccoli
- Asparagus
- Tomatoes
- Zucchini
- Whole grains
- Seafood
- Integral rice
- Sunflower seeds
- Eggs

Chapter 10

Medicinal plants

Plants can be used as medicines to prevent autoimmune diseases, lower and control glucose and to increase insulin sensitivity. Traditional Chinese medicine and Indian ayurveda have used the healing power of plants to struggle with diseases without prejudice of side effects, as well as with the advantage of getting multiple benefits for the organism. As an example, cinnamon helps lower blood glucose, and is also extremely effective in increasing the body's defenses.

Beneficial plants for diabetic people:

- **Green tea:** this has a substance called epigallocatechin gallate, which is an herb that stimulates the production of insulin. The presence of the beneficial components is not too high, so it is necessary to take between one and two liters a day of green tea.

- **Ginseng:** It should be consumed as an extract. Its effect is to increase insulin sensitivity, so the body takes advantage of it in a more efficient way.

- **Guarumbo leaves:** its effect is similar to the drug metformin, which is used to control type 2 diabetes; it reduces blood glucose and increases insulin sensitivity.

- **Ginger:** this root has fabulous effects for the digestive system. It is useful in type 2 diabetes because reduces the glucose in blood. The recommended dose is half a teaspoon before breakfast. The infusion of natural ginger is also very beneficial.

- **Fenugreek:** it decreases the presence of glucose in the blood and stimulates the production of insulin.

- **Eucalyptus:** An infusion of eucalyptus reduces blood glucose levels. The leaf of this tree helps in the process of glycogenogenesis, which implies the storage of glucose by the body so that it does not remain in the blood and damages the organs and nerves, but is released according to the demand of the organism.

- **Cranberry leaves:** they are equipped with a component called myrtiline, which has the same function as insulin: make the cell absorb glucose.

- **Berberine:** this plant fulfills the four functions that help control diabetes. First, it makes the liver to produce less glucose, also improves insulin sensitivity and, therefore, stimulates glucose uptake and finally reduces blood sugar levels.

- **Cinnamon:** it helps metabolize glucose and produce insulin. It should be consumed in moderate quantities, since it is very strong. It is an excellent seasoning for desserts and infusions.

- **Black curry:** this is a powerful herb with properties to protect the cardiovascular system and the liver. When consumed in small amounts at meals, the blood sugar level can be reduced by half.

- **Curcumin:** it protects the joints and the heart. The curcumin present in this spice reduces blood glucose. A pinch a day is recommended, either at meals or as a complement to other infusions.

- **Wereke:** the root of this plant has the effect of reducing blood sugar levels.

- **Wild gymnema:** the gymnemic acid presented in it stimulates the production of insulin by the pancreas.

- **Grape skin:** it contains procyanidin which helps the body to metabolize glucose correctly. Apart from that, it stimulates the pancreas to produce insulin.

Chapter 11

Endorsed products for diabetic people

The supermarket does not have to be a banned place for diabetic people. The associations and federations for diabetics located in different countries have endorsed the consumption of certain products. Next, you will find a compilation of them:

Splenda: this is a sweetener that allows you to reduce carbohydrates from sugar because it is made with sucralose. It comes in various presentations, which are adapted to the use that you want to give them, and can vary from sweetening a drink to preparing a dessert. There is a 100% natural option called Splenda Naturals Stevia.

Oleic oil: it is 100% natural and made from safflower seeds. It is ideal to complement meals without health risks

D'Gari jellies: the version for diabetics is light. There is also a line of drinks for diabetics of this same brand.

Sweet life: They are sweet lollipops of several flavors. You can find creamy or watery versions. Its flavors include honey-lemon, watermelon with chili, cherry, tangerine and mango with pineapple.

Stevia: every serving only has 3.7 calories. Use steviol glycosides to sweeten without increasing blood glucose.

Salmas: these are perfect for a healthy dessert; they are baked corn toast without fat or cholesterol.

McCormick jams: the label should say **sugar free**. It comes in the flavors of strawberry and red fruits. It is an excellent option, both for its health benefits and for its taste and consistency. It has pieces of fruit to keep the traditional format.

The Sevillanas: they are wafers, lollipops and glories sweetened with isomalt, a polyalcohol that does not affect blood sugar levels.

Don't Worry: They are sugar and fat free meringues. As their name says: there is nothing to worry about. The sandwich presentation is practical and easy to take everywhere.

Larin Chocolate: chocolate has lots of benefits to health, when consumed moderately. That is why Nestlé launched its Larin without sugar, so that diabetic people are not far from good and delicious desserts.

Charles V: it is a version of Nestle, it's a classic chocolate **sugar free**. It is sweetened with isomalt, which is a new ingredient from beet.

Bimbo bread: it is a version **zero** available for diabetic people. It comes natural or toasted and has no sugar or fat.

Prema jelly: you have to look for the **sugar free** version, this can be prepared in water or milk.

Chantilly Chanty Wip: There is a sugar-free version, which allows you to enjoy lots of desserts such as whipped cream. It has no sugar, but it does not mean that it does not contain fat or cholesterol. Therefore, its consumption should be moderate and spaced. The advantage is that it maintains the original flavor of the product.

Danone Vitaline: these are Greek style yogurts. We must look for those which **are free of sugar**, they are creamy and also to drink.

Chapter 12

Alternative therapies for managing diabetes

Apart from following a traditional treatment with our personal doctor, we also have the option of taking alternative therapies to prevent and control diabetes. Moreover, when treating diabetes, these therapies control and prevent consequences and associated diseases.

Alternative therapies

Plants medicinal treatment: as we see in the previous chapters, taking herbs, roots and spices can be very helpful to control diabetes. This is a simple and homemade way to treat this disease, as it does not have contraindications and does not go against traditional medical treatments.

Homeopathy: based on the principle of similarity, homeopathic drugs act to treat the symptoms of a specific illness. This alternative therapy uses substances dissolved in water our alcohol. This particular method affirms that could cause the symptoms in healthy people, so that it could remove them in those people who are truly sick.

Ozone therapy: despite the benefit of controlling diabetes, the use of ozone gives a lot of advantages to cellular system, improving its functions. It consists in apply ozone to patients through oils, creams, glass bell, plastic chambers, and also injections. By boosting the cell's functions, it helps to take glucose from the blood to inside the cells. It is not indicated for people that had had heart attacks, pregnant women, or patients allergic.

Acupuncture: it helps to palliate diabetes symptoms by improve in metabolic functions, so as to avoid the progression of the disease. Acupuncture is part from the traditional Chinese medicine and also Japanese. It consists in introducing small needles into the subcutaneous tissue in strategic zones in the body, which activate a natural mechanism to relieve an illness

Bach flowers: this therapy is bases in indentifying emotional and psychological causes among diseases. It says that those who suffer from a disease, such as diabetes, have a deep bitterness and expend their lives thing on "things that could have happened if...", but they did not reach it. This method offers cures to control emotions, and avoid their negative effects on the pancreas. There are some recipes advisable for diabetics, such as: Cherry Plum, Holly, Crab Apple, Mustard, and Honey suckle and Star of Bethlehem.

All these therapies can be use to struggle with diabetes and its associated diseases. In any case, it is advisable to ask your doctor about this new alternative treatment and see if it matches with your clinical condition as a complement for managing.

Self-help groups for people with diabetes

It is very common that a person who suffers from a disease feels that he/she is lonely. To avoid this, there are some self-help groups that can be helpful to get emotional support. There, people with the same disease have the chance to talk and share experience, it works as a therapy.

Self-help groups can be face-to-face, or using the new technologies, it is also possible to get in contact by internet.

Many countries have their own self-help groups. What truly counts is find the moment appropriated to get in contact and assist. Every person is different, so it is important that the patient and his/her family talk about when start visiting a self-help group. A general advice is to wait for a period where is kind of a "window" between the diagnoses and the start of the treatment.

The first step is to accept that we will have to live with this illness. Once that information is accepted for our minds, the next step can be going into a self-help group that can be "a partner" to face this new moment in life, where lots of changes will come in lifestyles and things that we were used to.

There are some websites for support patients with diabetes, they offered advices and interesting news. These are:

- **Spanish Diabetic Federation (FEDE)**
- **Diabetes channel**
- **Center for the innovation of childhood diabetes (CIDI)**
- **Families with diabetes**
- **People who live with diabetes**

Educational therapy in diabetes

It is known as ETD, it is very important because the educational therapy is part of the management of diabetes. This is an attempt to raise awareness about the importance of taking care of ourselves. It involves family and some practices that help the patient to get control of his/her life to reach changes in lifestyle and habits that with improve diabetes. The objective is teaching the patient and his/her family that there are attitudes which can improve life to have more control of the disease.

Topic II

Obesity

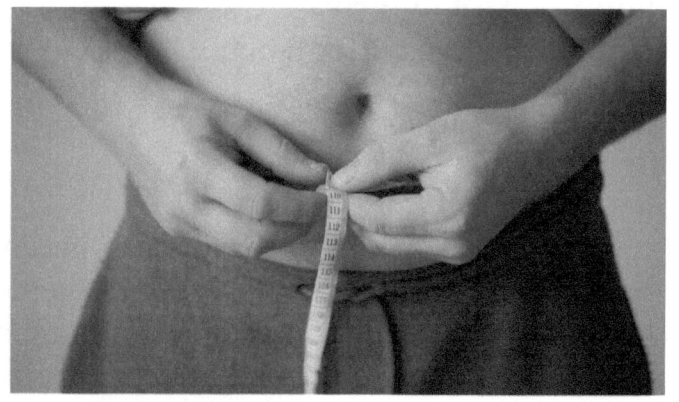

Chapter 1

Concept

Obesity is a chronic disease that, in most cases, can be prevented. It is the accumulation of excessive adipose tissues. Although adipose tissue plays a fundamental role in health because this is where energy is stored, when it grows excessively, it not only damages our aesthetics, but also compromises our health, since obesity is the fifth disease that involves risk of death worldwide. Obesity can be classified according to body mass index.

Obesity types according to BMI

The body mass index (BMI) is an indicator that determines the type of obesity suffered. We get it by finding the quotient between the person's weight and his height squared.

For example, if we take a person which height is 1,75m and his/her weight is 80 kg, the count is as follows:

$$80 \text{ kg} \div (1,70)^2 \text{ m} = 28 \text{ IMC kg/m}$$

According to BMI, obesity types are:

BMI

- **Normal weight:** 18,5 – 24,9
- **Overweight:** 25 - 29
- **Grade 1:** 30 - 34
- **Grade 2:** 35 – 39,9
- **Grade 3:** 40 – 49,9
- **Grade 4:** more than 50

Since obesity grade 1 starts a serious problem for health.

Android vs. Gynecoid Obesity

Other way to classified obesity is according to the distribution of adipose tissue. In this case we have two types, android and gynecoid obesity.

Android Obesity: fat is accumulated in the abdominal area, chest and face, so the person has an "apple appearance". This type of obesity can indicate diabetes and tends to cause cardiovascular diseases.

Gynecoid Obesity: fat accumulates excessively in the thighs and hips. Women are the most likely to develop it and usually lead to varicose veins or knee osteoarthritis.

Chapter 2

Most frequent causes

Obesity can appear because of many causes. Among these we found genetic aspects and diseases. Talking in general, the most common causes for obesity are:

Genetic: genes predispose to obesity, but they don't act along. If one of the parents is obese, the person has a 50% chance of being so, while if both parents are, the chance increases to 80%. As we see, there is a possibility but we also can avoid it. In cases of genetics, obesity appears if we eat a diet rich in sugars and saturated fats and if we do not practice physical exercise. The role of genes determines the appetite of a person, the amount and size of fat cells, the distribution of adipose tissue and the degree of calorie burning. That is, the metabolism is conditioned by genetics, but the metabolism is not everything in terms of obesity. It only indicates that we will have to make a greater effort to stay in a healthy weight.

Lifestyle and habits: eating and exercise habits are decisive in the issue of obesity. Avoiding this disease depends largely on staying active and eating foods that, far from generating adipose tissue, act by absorbing fats and eliminating them from the body.

Medications: as side effects of some medications, there is obesity. The reason for which some drugs make us get weight is because some alter the metabolism, others increase appetite, others simply accumulate fat in the body and others produce fluid retention. These are antidepressants, beta blockers (they treat hypertension and heart problems), steroids and antipsychotic.

Endocrine causes: fatty tissue depends on hormonal secretion, so some diseases which affect endocrine system can lead to obesity. The most commons are hyperinsulinemia (a level of insulin in blood higher than normal) and an increased secretion of leptine (obesity hormone).

Other endocrine causes that can lead to obesity are:

Resistance to the action of insulin: it is the inability of insulin in the blood to do its function of keeping blood sugar within certain levels because the tissues don't respond to it.

Polycystic ovary: Up to 60% of women suffering from polycystic ovarian syndrome (PCOS) suffer from obesity. This syndrome doesn't release the mature ovum into the fallopian tubes, so they accumulate in the ovaries generating endless disorders.

Hypothyroidism: occurs when the thyroid does not secrete enough T4 and T3 hormones, they're responsible for various functions in the body, for example, the metabolism of food for proper fat burning.

Cushing: Cushing's syndrome occurs when the body produces too much cortisol, the stress hormone, for very long periods. It can happen when the person suffers from emotional or psychological stress, as well as due to taking corticosteroid medications.

Hypogonadism: it's when men do not produce enough testosterone. This deficiency can occur in the fetal stage, before the onset of puberty or in the adult stage.

Gigantism: due to the excessive presence of growth hormone (GH), the body grows excessively.

Acromegaly: it's when the growth hormone (GH) is secreted in excessive amounts in adulthood. There is an exaggerated growth of the hands and feet. The difference with gigantism is that in acromegaly, long bones can no longer grow because the growth points are ossified.

Chapter 3

Most common symptoms

There are some cases where due to the conformation of the body, it can be difficult to realize if we have exceeded the limit of overweight and we are on the side of obesity. If we have not done the calculation of our body mass index and we are experiencing at least two of these symptoms constantly, it is a good time to do start being concerned about it.

Weight gain: it is the first symptom. It's indicating that obesity is coming. We can noticed by the way of clothes fit us, and testing our weight.

Acanthosis nigricans: is the thickening and darkening of the skin in the areas of joints or folds, such as elbows, knees, neck, knuckles and armpits.

Stretch marks: when there is an abrupt stretch in the skin, small grooves appear on the skin that may be lighter or darker than the skin tone. Their appearance can be distressing for the person, but they are not harmful or painful.

Menstrual disorders: amenorrhea is the most common, which consists in the absence of menstrual cycles for prolonged periods.

Knee pain: due to weight, the knee joint suffers and eventually starts having problems to move, walk and hurts.

Other symptoms in obesity:

- Excessive sweating
- Troubles to sleep
- More risk to suffer from infections
- Back and joint pain
- Depression
- Fatigue
- Heat intolerance
- Shortness of breath

Chapter 4

Associated diseases

The human body is kind of a large interconnected network. If something happens in one part of it, several others are affected. In the case of obesity, this can lead to diseases and consequences that are detailed below:

Hypertension: the reasons why obesity causes high blood pressure are because it increases sodium retention in the body, which leads to fluid retention. On the other hand, the heart must work harder to pump the same volume of blood.

Irritable bowel: it's a digestive disorder whose symptoms are constipation and diarrhea, without apparent cause. The abdomen swells and becomes distended, generating persistent pain.

Gastroesophageal reflux: it is caused because the esophageal sphincter loses strength due to pressure inside the abdomen.

Renal impairment: when body mass increases, it also does the risk of chronic kidney disease. The organism performs a more intense filtration to compensate for metabolic demand, so over time this can lead to kidney disease.

Renal and vesicular lithiasis: a high body mass index in people leads to develop renal lithiasis. Almost 60% of people with kidney or bladder stones are obese.

Coronary heart disease: overweight decreases fibrinolysis, which increases the risk of thrombosis, a factor associated with heart disease.

Diabetes: obesity causes resistance to the action of insulin, which is the main pathological change to develop type 2 diabetes. The body cannot use insulin, so there's a high level of sugar in blood.

High cholesterol: the presence high level of bad cholesterol (LDL) in blood is a risk that occurs because of sedentary lifestyle. It is not obesity in itself that generates it, but the lack of physical exercise due to the effort involved when suffering from obesity.

Moreover, obesity can increase the risk of cancer in a 50% and may causes psychological diseases, such as anxiety and depression.

Chapter 5

Consequences

Hepatic steatosis: also known as fatty liver, this is a disease that leads the liver to accumulate fat. Another cause is excessive alcohol intake. However, it's more likely to occur due to an unhealthy diet that also leads to obesity. It is prevented and controlled by eating foods with omega 3 fatty acids, such as blue fish. It is necessary to keep cholesterol levels under control, do aerobic exercise and be very careful with diets, since the loss of more than 4 kilos per month could aggravate this condition.

Metabolic syndrome: it is caused by sugar blood in levels higher than normal. It is characterized by the accumulation of adipose tissue around the waist. It is prevented and controlled through diet based on fruits and vegetables, lean proteins and whole grains. You should avoid salt in meals and do not to consume saturated fats. Aerobic exercise must be daily and a minimum of thirty minutes per day. You must not smoke.

Hyperuricemia: this is the excess uric acid in blood. It is prevented and controlled by reducing the consumption of red meat and liver, chocolate and canned foods. It is essential to drink two litters of water per day, since the purines responsible for uric acid are eliminated in the urine.

Acrocordones: these are small tumors that form in places where the skin has folds and friction occurs. They are often confused with warts. The prevention consists in losing weight, since this is how the skin will rub less. They can be mitigated and even disappear with apple cider vinegar, castor oil or pineapple juice. We only have to choose one of these three components and apply it three times a day until it disappears or minimizes.

Osteoarthrosis: when the joint cartilage that protects the joints between the bones is lost, they begin to rub against each other and wear out, causing pain, deformation in the joints and loss of range of motion. Maintaining an adequate body weight is one of the best ways to prevent it, as well as educating yourself about postures when walking or resting. When it hurts, applying a heat source will relieve the discomfort, while if it becomes inflamed, it is convenient to apply an ice pack.

Chapter 6

Treatments

Conventional treatment for obesity is based in three steps: diet changes so as to reduce calories intake, aerobic and anaerobic physical exercise to increase the use of calories, and changes in lifestyle to control a compulsive behavior when eating.

Drugs and surgeries are part of the treatment against obesity as a plan B. These always need to be advised by a specialist who examines the clinical condition of the patient, and who knows the right indication and side effects of the drug and surgeries.

Medications

Medications for obesity are indicated in people with BMI higher than 30 kg / m^2, that is, with type I obesity, or overweight (BMI> 27 kg / m^2) who have comorbidities associated (diabetes, hypertension, dyslipidemias) and who have not responded to the initial measures of diet, exercises and changes in behavior, having met them exactly. The mechanism of action by which these drugs act can be of two types:

(1) To inhibit appetite, that is, they are anorexigenic medications; or

(2) To reduce the absorption of carbohydrates and fats through the inhibition of the enzymatic proteins of the intestine that help to incorporate food into the body (pancreatic lipases)

When you adopt diet measures and exercise, the body's internal metabolism resists such changes by making physiological adaptations that seek to prevent weight reduction, for example, increased appetite. That is why many times, weight that is lost tends to be recovered. At this point the drugs act, decrease the action of these physiological mechanisms of our body that resist weight loss, so that diet and exercise are effective and the changes are maintained in the long term.

Drug therapy has been effective when in a period of 12 weeks after its use, combined with diet and exercise, 5% of body weight has been lost. If this objective has not been achieved, adherence to treatment should be reviewed as it is possible that some stage is not being met exactly.

A question that is always present is: *is it necessary to take medication?* The answer depends a lot on the clinical situation of the patient. Medications do not have any direct effect on weight loss, all they do is help to maintain the metabolic changes that are generated with diet and exercise, so without changes in lifestyle the medications do not work. As we see, diet and exercise are the pillars of obesity treatment. Some drugs for the treatment of obesity are:

- **Derivatives of amphetamines (Phentermine, Diethylpropion)**: they act on central nervous system to reduce appetite. They are recommended for short periods of time usually 12 weeks.
- **Orlistat:** this is one of the most used. It blocks the action of gastro-pancreatic lipase to prevent the absorption of fats in the intestine. It can be used for longer periods, up to 1 year.
- **Topiramate:** this is a drug mainly used to treat epilepsy, but also acts on the inhibition of appetite at the central level. It can be used for a long time.
- **Bupropion:** this drug is used to treat depression and tobacco addiction and decreases appetite. It can be used for a long time.

The drug must be chosen by a specialist who needs to consider the clinical condition of the patient. Some side effects are vomiting, diarrhea, constipation, dry mouth, palpitations, high blood pressure. This cannot be taken by children or pregnant women.

Surgeries

There are surgeries which remove the excess of fatty tissue, change appetite and make people eat less.

Bariatric surgery: the most common is the gastric baipas. It consists in a combination of restrictive surgery, to reduce the size of the stomach by an elastic band, and a malabsortive surgery, whose function is to make food reach the small intestine faster so that it won't be absorbed completely. This surgery not only eliminates obesity, but also the risks of developing diseases derived from it.

Bariatric surgery is recommended when any diet, exercise or medication treatment has worked, so there is a danger of life due to complications associated with obesity.

Possible side effects of this surgery are vomiting, gallstones, diarrhea, increased gas, excessive sweating, nutritional deficiencies and dizziness.

Aesthetic: the most common are tummy tuck (in the abdomen), mammoplasty (in the breasts), and surgeries to remove fatty tissue in arms and thighs. These surgeries are not recommended to treat obesity, since without proper changes in lifestyle, weight is recovered. The way to make it more effective is to lose weight and exercise at the same time. What these surgeries do is to remove excess skin due to stretching caused by obesity.

Liposculpture: this is a procedure that allows the removal of excess fat in localized areas. It is recommended after having achieved an ideal weight, because at that point you can appreciate better remaining adipose tissue. The area to be treated is anesthetized and a cannula is introduced to inject tumescent fluid, which releases the fat. With the help of another cannula, that fat is aspirated. The expectations that we have about this surgery are very important, since they do not promise the perfect body, but the improvement of the silhouette. The side effects are mainly transient, since they have to do with swelling, pain, discoloration and bruising of the skin. Since this intervention does not stretch the skin completely, it is contraindicated for patients with a marked overweight or very aging skin.

Chapter 7

Physical activity

Exercise possibilities and consequences

One of the solutions to overweight is exercise. However, mobility possibilities represent a problem when this disease is suffered. Therefore, we have to keep in mind that the ranges of movement and the exercises are not the same for people with normal weight.

The purpose is reducing the BMI to lose weight, but the exercise routine needs to be designed for each person with obesity according to his/her possibilities.

The back is a weak point for obese people, so it will be necessary to improve muscle tone in this area and counteract working the abdominal part, including the oblique. Although aerobic exercise is essential, it must be complemented with resistance, elasticity and flexibility routines.

Diseases and consequences

Complications associated with exercise during obesity are related to muscle, joint and cardiovascular system injuries.

We should not force our heart to the fullest, as this could be dangerous. So, we must exercise in a moderate and constant manner. When we add weight to our resistance routines, we must do it very gradually and moderately. Finally, warming and stretching are essential to avoid injuries.

Aerobic routines

Any of these aerobic exercises needs to be practice every day for at least 25 minutes continuous.

- Treadmill.
- March simulating waking but raising your knees as much as possible.
- Raise the knee to touch the opposite elbow. It should be repeated 10 times each side.
- Moderated aerobic class with choreography.
- Extend the arms cross and raise the right knee to the right elbow and the left to the left.

Resistance routines

These are practiced after some heating exercises during 5 minutes.

- **Squats with rotation of shoulders:** it is about putting the feet a little more apart than the width of the shoulders and moving backwards as if we wanted to sit down. When we return, we bring the flexed arms to chest height and rotate the body to the side. In the next squat we turn it to the other. We repeat thirty times.

- **Rowing:** with the feet slightly apart, we bring the chest at 45° with respect to the floor, we extend the arms forward, each with a dumbbell of 3 kilos; we place the palms up and bring the elbows back and return the extended arms forward. We do three sets of twenty repetitions.

- **Side support:** we lie on a firm table supporting the forearm and holding the body in a straight line, but leaning towards the table.

Elasticity routines

After resistance exercise we go to practice elasticity:

- **Chest expansion:** lie with the face to the floor, place your hands at shoulder height, stretch your arms and bring your body back. The head should be straight, not backward. Hold it twenty seconds, go back to the floor and repeat twice more.

- **Leg elasticity:** lie on your back, bring one knee to your chest and extend your leg up. Leave it at 90° from the floor and with the knee well stretched.

Do it again with the other leg. You should do 20 seconds of each exercise and repeat three times with each leg.

Flexibility routines

At the end of the resistance exercises, we should do a flexibility routine:

- We separate the feet a little and take a step forward with one of them. We raise the arm of the leg that is behind and turn the trunk towards the side of the leg that is ahead. We wait twenty seconds and go to the other side.

- We separate the feet a little more than the width of the shoulders and tilt the trunk to the side. We help each other by bringing the arm to the side we lean and the other forward. You can also do this sitting on the floor and with your legs apart.

Chapter 8

Dietary measures

Low calorie diet

A low calorie diet consists of decreasing the amounts of calories we consume. At first it seems to be the most logical and mathematical solution to obesity: fewer calories = lower body mass index, but the factors that come into play make it an enemy potential of obesity.

By consuming fewer calories, we feel colder and the circulatory system suffers. On the other hand, digestion spends fewer calories, so we assimilate more food while eating.

Finally, physical activity is reduced instinctively. In the absence of energy, the brain orders to stop movement so that the body does not finish losing the few reserves it has.

Also a low calorie diet can harm the body, so that it is necessary to complement it with the increase of proteins and lipids.

So the key is a balanced diet and exercise daily.

Fad diets

Fad diets are usually followed for a short period of time: between a week and a month. The goal is to drastically lose weight. However, due to the lack of nutrients they present, they become unviable in the long term. Therefore, it is impossible not to generate the rebound effect after them.

They are based on few ingredients whose slimming properties have recently been discovered. The only case in which we recommend them is when we already have a planed diet that we will follow after it and as long as the diet begins with physical exercise and this continues indefinitely after the diet.

It is not surprising that these diets can make you lose 15 kg in a month, but you can recover even more when returning to your routine. Another factor is that they produce a strong bad mood and irritability for making us deprived of eating lots of tasty things, such as chocolate.

Diets according to glycemic index

Diets according to the glycemic index are those on which we base the diet on food according to its influence on blood sugar levels. Foods that have carbohydrates get a number, which will depend on how much they can increase blood sugar.

This is a diet that counts carbohydrates and calories to avoid exceeding the ideal limit and thus keep blood sugar controlled. The objectives you can achieve through this count are to have a healthy diet, lose weight and prevent diabetes.

The glycemic index is divided into three categories:

- Low glycemic index: 1 to 55
- Medium glycemic index: 56 to 69
- High glycemic index: 70 and up

As for food, these are divided into:

- Low glycemic load: 1 to 10
- Medium glycemic load: 11 to 19
- High glycemic load: 20 onwards

Low glycemic load foods: green vegetables, carrots, red beans, chickpeas and lentils.
Medium glycemic load foods: bananas, pineapple, raisins, oats, sweet corn and rye bread.
High glycemic load foods: potatoes and white bread

Recommended foods

- Cereals
- Integral rice
- Potatoes
- Integral food (not processed)
- Fruits
- Vegetables and legumes

- Water
- Lean broth
- Infusions
- Natural juices
- Legumes
- Olive oil

Ways of cooking most recommended

- Baked
- Steamed
- Boiled
- Sweetened with natural sweeteners
- Sautéed with altoleic oil
- Lean
- Grilled

It is recommend all kind of food but no fried, or those which ingredients are too much fatty.

Menu examples

Breakfast

- 1 fruit
- 1 cup of cereal
- 100 g of cheese

Lunch

- 1 Portion of integral rice with vegetables
- 1 cup of lean broth
- 1 fruit or dairy product without sugar

Snack

- 2 slices of bread toasted with jam without sugar
- 1 cup of coffee with milk without sugar

Dinner

- 3 pieces of baked broccoli
- 1 Portion of beet and carrot raw salad with olive oil and vinegar.
- 1 fruit

As snacks: fruits, rice crackers, lean cheese and sugar-free cereal bars are recommended, just one or two in the case of rice crackers. In the case of cheese it is enough with 100 gr.

Attractive and healthy culinary recipes

Fresh tuna with mushrooms and peppers

- 2 fresh tuna fillets
- 1 onion
- ¼ of pepper

- 10 mushrooms
- Altoleic oil

Cut the vegetables in julienne and the mushrooms and put them in the oil. When ready, add the tuna steaks and cook by both sides until they are ready. You can season with spices to your liking.

Napolitan lentils burgers

- 2 cups of cooked lentils
- ½ cup of rye flour
- 2 slices of cheese
- 2 slices of tomato

Mash the lentils well drained and season them to taste. Add the rye flour, mixture until you have a homogeneous paste. Take to the refrigerator for two hours. Take it out and form two hamburgers. Put them on the non-stick iron without oil. Finally, add a cheese to each and the tomato slice.

How to avoid "the rebound"

The rebound is the forced effect of an inappropriate diet. Therefore, avoiding is far from taking those fat diets which promises lose more than 10 kg in a week.

What you need to do is to change life habits: eat healthy, drop sugar, exercise every day (ideally two hours, although thirty minutes is enough) and drink a minimum of two liters of water a day. These habits will allow us to lose weight gradually and stay in it.

Chapter 9

Vitamins and minerals

Vitamins and minerals that cannot be out of an anti-obesity diet

Our metabolism is responsible, in part, for obesity. It is not just what we eat, but what our body does with it once we have eaten. A slow metabolism means that the smallest food intake is assimilated and stored as an energy reserve.

We can avoid that. There is a wide list of vitamins and minerals which can improve metabolic functions by boosting them and helping us to lose weight.

Vitamins

- Vitamin A
- Vitamin C
- Vitamin D
- Vitamin E

Minerals

- Calcium
- Magnesium

Food rich in vitamin A

- Milk
- Butter
- Cheddar
- Broccoli
- Cabbage
- Carrots
- Spinach
- Mango
- Fruit melon
- Chicken
- Turkey
- Meat
- Fish

Food rich in vitamin C

- Orange
- Tangerine
- Grapefruit
- Lemon
- Kiwi
- Parsley
- Red pepper
- Broccoli
- Strawberry
- Khaki
- Basil
- Papaya

Food rich in vitamin D

It is important to know that 30% of the vitamin D that our body needs comes from food, and the rest 70% depends on the sun. When we expose to sun our body is able to produce vitamin D. So, try to expose to sun just for few minutes a day. Some foods which have vitamin D are:

- Sardines
- Tuna
- Salmon
- Fish oil
- Milk
- Cheese
- Yogurt
- Butter
- Wheat germ
- Mushrooms
- Avocado

Food rich in vitamin E

- Legumes
- Eggs
- Olive oil
- Sunflower oil
- Integral cereals
- Avocado

- Papaya
- Milk
- Butter
- Nuts
- Chia seeds
- Sunflower seeds
- Green vegetables
- Blue fish

Food rich in calcium

- Cheese
- Yogurt
- Milk
- Butter
- Asparagus
- Spinach
- Broccoli
- Chard
- Cabbage
- Sardines
- Salmon
- Seafood

Food rich in magnesium

- Green Vegetables
- Nuts
- Cherries

- Plantain
- Legumes
- Cocoa
- Integral cereals
- Fish

Chapter 10

Medicinal Plants

Beneficial Medicinal Plants

Plants recommended to struggle with obesity are those which help the body to burn fats, increase the use of calories, avoid the conversion of glucose into fat and keep us without hunger.

Burn fats

- Green tea
- Yerba mate
- Guarana
- Green coffee
- Fennel
- Dandelion
- Chicory
- Black radish

Reduce hunger

- California poppy
- Valerian
- Plantago
- Glucomannan

- Spirulina

Reduce the absorption of food

- Garciniacambogia
- Horsetail
- Nettle

Increase the use of calories

- Birch
- Thistle

Reduce the resistance to insulin

- Cinnamon
- Wild gymnema
- Glucomannan
- Ginseng

Chapter 11

Natural supplements

Companies such as Life have dedicated their lives to research in health issues. To reflect this, they created natural supplements to counteract harmful effects that the body receives. All of them share a number of ingredients in common and work to eliminate obesity. It is very important to know them, before deciding to consume.

Caffeine

By increasing the cardiac effect, it accelerates the metabolism. It has a strong oxidative effect on fats. On the other hand, resistance increases, which is very beneficial for people in a progressive exercise program.

Whey protein

Its action is to increase muscle mass, and so stimulates the loss of fat, since the muscle feeds on it. When consuming it, we are likely to gain weight, but we are changing fat for muscle, which is healthy.

Vitamin D

It helps in the absorption of calcium from food and, therefore, burns excess fat in the body.

Chitosan

It has the power to absorb and purify the fats that enter our body through food. Therefore, it reduces body mass and decreases abdominal swelling.

Hydroxycitric acid

It is present in the garciniacambogia plant and its effect is to absorb the accumulated fat in the abdomen, in the liver and under the skin.

Presentations of weight loss supplements

Diuretics: these activate renal function and prevent fluid retention. The body loses volume thanks to the purification of the liquids stored.

Meal substitutes: they have the necessary nutrients to replace one of the four meals of the day. These are designed to replace light meals, they are recommended for eating as a snack or dinner.

Satiating: these have soluble and insoluble fibers. Fiber doubles its size by absorbing the water present in the stomach and gives the sensation of eating much more than we have actually eaten.

Laxatives: you have to be very careful with these products to lose weight. The laxative helps to eliminate waste, which does not mean that it thins, but deflates. If it is taken frequently even if it is not needed, it does not allow the intestine to absorb nutrients, then it ends up making the body sick. Laxatives should not be used for weight loss.

Fat burners: their function is to stimulate fat metabolism, which means sending an order to the body to use the deposits of fat more quickly. Sometimes it happens that the body does not react and does not use these reserves. This is why burners are highly effective in these cases.

Chapter 12

Alternative therapies

There are some alternatives with are 100% naturals to control obesity. These aren't harmful because don't act against the effect of nutrients, they work using plants, natural resources and meditation. The better known are:

Behavioral therapies

It is about inducing a state of calm through the control of breathing, muscle tension-relaxation-heaviness through the awareness of each muscle and mindfulness training, which is about directing energy to each part of the body to achieve effects of cold, heat, warmth and pressure, among others.

Stress control

Aromatherapy: this alternative therapy has many uses, for example stress control. By mixing the right aromas, permanent relaxation can be generated to achieve body-mind-spirit harmony.

Laughter therapy: it is a very modern technique and is based on the laughter tested to generate spontaneous. Believe in the contagious effect of laughter, it is about making the participants laugh. It releases tensions and leads to the cure of diseases associated with bitterness and stress.

Breathing: this technique is about to make controlled inspirations and exhalations to lower levels of stress and tension.

Music therapy: by using the notes indicated for each case, music works as a great therapist. Blood pressure is reduced, hormonal levels are regulated and heart rate is controlled.

Massages: by the correct stimulation of strategic zones, the state of adequate relaxation is achieved.

Relaxation therapies

- **Meditation:** Through focused attention techniques, silence, proper body posture and controlled breathing, stress is taken out of the body.

- **Progressive relaxation:** it can be practiced at any time and in any place. You have to start from above or below and continue in order. It consists of stressing the muscles of a part of the body to immediately relax them.

- **Biofeedback:** in this, sensors are placed in the body which helps to see the different rhythms and body values. When they are determined, you have to change your mind to modify them.

- **Taichi:** when working on balance and concentration through slow and controlled movements, the tension caused by stress is removed.

- **Yoga:** forced yoga postures generate body control have a very positive metabolic change. One of these effects is to eliminate stress.

Anxiety Control

Anxiety can be controlled by using herbs, homeopathy treatments or Bach flowers. These are natural therapies so we need to be patient and wait for a few weeks to see the results in our body.

Depression Control

In depression are involved lots of internal and external factors. The treatment may need antidepressant foods such as eggs, nuts, chocolate, and also practice exercise frequently, dance, and do activities that we enjoy. Trying to share more with family and friends is also a great therapy to control depression.

Control carbohydrates addiction

Carbohydrates cannot be excluded of diet because they are the main source of energy. What we could do is control their intake as follow:

- **Reduce the intake of carbohydrates**
- **Add to diet polyunsaturated fats (walnuts, peneaut butter)**
- **Avoid starchy carbohydrates for dinner**

Compulsion Control

To control compulsive alimentary behavior it is needed the help of professionals such as:

- **Psychologist**
- **Psychiatrist**
- **Nutritionist**
- **Physician**

Body image

When someone suffers from body image distortion, the most effective treatments are:

- **Behavior and cognitive therapies**
- **Medications that increases serotonine (antidepressants)**

Hedonistic eater

It is the kind of person who looks for delighting through food. It is not just because of the food itself, but the sensations that it causes. On the other hand, since hedonism is associated with well-being, it is a person who eats to get healthy through food. So, he/she chooses foods that are rich and healthy at the same time.

Topic III

Thyroid Gland Diseases

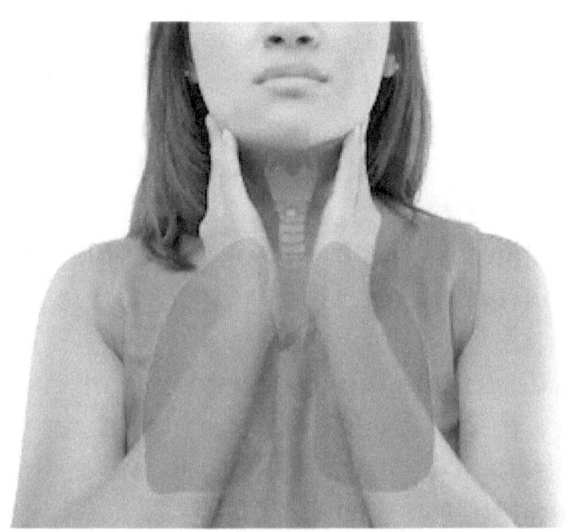

Chapter 1

Concept

In our neck there is a gland which looks like a butterfly and it is called thyroid. Its function is to produce hormones for the proper functioning of systems and body organs, these hormones are important for the dynamic of metabolism.

When the thyroid gland is affected by diseases or other conditions, this impacts various systems in our body. The symptoms can be imperceptible at the beginning, such as becoming more sensitive to cold, but then they become very serious, as in the case of extreme obesity or extreme thinness, both without an explanation related to food or physical exercise.

In order to determine the existence of a thyroid failure it is necessary to do some tests, such as determination of blood levels of T4 hormone. Sometimes a biopsy may be requested too.

Kinds of thyroid gland diseases

The most frequent diseases affecting thyroid gland are: hyperthyroidism, hypothyroidism, Hashimoto's thyroiditis and Goiter.

Hypothyroidism: it occurs when the thyroid gland does not produce enough thyroid hormone, so the body cannot perform relevant functions in its systems. It is more common in women than in men and usually manifests after sixty years old.

Hyperthyroidism: we are in the presence of this pathology when the thyroid is too active and, therefore, produces an excess of thyroid hormone. It may appear due to an excessive consumption of iodine, thyroid nodules or simply because of gender and age, since women are the most likely to develop this problem, as well as people over sixty years old.

Hashimoto's thyroiditis: It is also known as chronic lymphocytic thyroiditis and occurs when the immune system attacks the thyroid gland cells.

Goiter: it is the enlargement of the thyroid gland, which manifests through the swelling of the neck. The most common cause of goiter is the lack of iodine; the gland is enlarged in an attempt to absorb all possible iodine from our diet. Without enough iodine, the thyroid cannot produce enough thyroid hormone.

Chapter 2

Most frequent causes

The most frequent causes for thyroid gland diseases are:

Autoimmunity: autoimmune diseases, such as rheumatoid arthritis, celiac disease, type 1 diabetes, Addison's disease, pernicious anemia, multiple sclerosis or in cases of Turner or Down syndrome, or bipolar disease, may lead to hyper or hypothyroidism.

Iodine deficiency: a diet low in iodine can cause hypothyroidism.

Premenopause: hormonal changes that happen at this stage can trigger thyroid problems.

Genetic: there is a high probability of hypo or hyperthyroidism if our parents have had it, especially if it was due to Hashimoto or Graves disease.

Hyperactive nodules: thyroid nodules can lead to excessive production of T4.

Thyroiditis: is the inflammation of the gland, which is caused by pregnancy, autoimmunity or for reasons that are not well-known.

Smoking: the thiocyanates present in tobacco can produce goiter.

To avoid thyroid gland diseases it is advisable to choose organic cleaning products and cosmetics, because many of these products contain substances that negatively affect hormone production. Stress is another cause of thyroid diseases, so we should avoid it as much as possible. It is evident that sometimes it is not possible to work less, but we can control the way in which the problems related to this aspect of our life affect us.

Chapter 3

Most frequent symptoms

According to the type of disease affecting the thyroid gland, its symptoms can vary.

Hypothyroidism

- Tiredness
- Daytime sleepiness
- Dry skin
- Overweight
- Forgetfulness
- Fatigue
- Cold sensitivity
- Weakness
- Hoarseness
- Constipation
- Slow heart rate
- Facial swelling
- Thyroid swelling (goiter)
- High Cholesterol
- Joint pain and swelling
- Depression

Hyperthyroidism

- Palpitations
- Nervousness, irritability, anxiety
- Tremors
- Weight loss
- Nightmares
- Fatigue
- Increased appetite
- Increased perspiration
- Heat sensitivity and suffocation
- Hair loss
- Menstrual disorders
- Diarrhea
- Breast growth in men
- Vomiting and nausea

Hashimoto's disease

- Symptoms can be similar to hypothyroidism or hyperthyroidism
- Small goiter
- Swollen tongue
- Brittle nails
- Menorrahagia (excessive bleeding during menstruation)
- Hair loss

Goiter

- It may have no symptoms
- Goiter
- Difficulty swallowing, breathing or speaking.
- Cough
- Sensation of tightness in the throat

Chapter 4

Associated diseases

When a thyroid gland disease starts, it can be followed by some other pathology, among these we have:

Irritable bowel: Hypothyroidism can cause intestinal diseases, such as gluten intolerance or problems associated with the irritable bowel. Therefore, certain foods, especially those that contain fibers, may cause discomfort.

Depression: one of the first tests that a doctor requests to study the onset of depression symptoms is thyroid function. If depression were due to this cause, antidepressant treatment wouldn't work; the hypothyroidism needs to be treated.

Fibromyalgia: there is an intense and persistent pain in skeletal muscles. It can be caused by a wide range of factors, among which is hypothyroidism.

Hypertension: the endocrine system, of which the thyroid is a part, is related to the appearance of secondary hypertension, this is when the cause is not the excessive sodium intake, lack of exercise or genetics.

Arthritis: hypothyroidism can cause pain related to this disease, as well as swelling of the joints present in the hands and feet.

Chapter 5

Consequences

Untreated thyroid disease can lead to consequences of extreme severity. That is why periodic monitoring is very important to treat thyroid problems that could cause the following:

Infertility: thyroid hormones interact with sex hormones. Therefore, they play a very important role in the maturation, release and fertilization of the ovules. A thyroid malfunction can lead from difficulty conceiving and to spontaneous abortions. Men also experience problems with their sperm, so infertility is not just a female problem. To help the management of this problem you can consume foods rich in iodine, including cow's milk, cheese, fish and eggs.

Sexual dysfunction: the physical and psychic disorders can affect sexuality. Some troubles are erectile dysfunction, premature ejaculation, lack of desire, aversion to sex, pain during sex and the inability to have orgasms. One of the best ways to prevent and solve this is through a fluid and effective communication with the couple. A thyroid disease can be one of the causes, so it is recommended to change diet and lifestyle to be healthy. Some medications, such as antidepressants and antihypertensive, affect too, so the recommendations are to look for a natural alternatives. Always eliminating the causes of diseases are the healthiest measures to take. For example, if you suffer from high blood pressure, the first thing is to eliminate is salt and do thirty minutes of aerobic exercise a day.

Dementia: when body chemistry derived from the endocrine system is altered, one of the possible consequences is the loss of faculties and mental function. It is essential to detect this pathology; otherwise, the brain damage could be permanent. Both high and low thyroid hormone levels can lead to this problem. To reverse hypothyroidism you can use dandelion tea or ginseng tea. In the case of hyperthyroidism, the intake of radish is recommended, either in salads or in the form of juice mixed with lemon.

Heart disease: while hypothyroidism directly affects the cardiovascular system, hyperthyroidism has a predisposition to cause atrial fibrillation, which is a serious arrhythmia.

Thyroid cancer: thyroid cancer is mainly due to genetics and factors such as radiation exposure in childhood. Because this last factor has a minimal incidence in its appearance, it is very difficult to prevent the disease. However, there are natural alternatives that help deal with treatments against this type of cancer. It is recommended to adopt the Mediterranean diet, which is based on orange and red vegetables, citrus fruits, green vegetables, red fruits and legumes, among other natural foods.

Chapter 6

Treatments

Medications

In the treatment of thyroid diseases, medications can be used to stimulate its function, when there is hypothyroidism, or to reduce its excessive activity when there is hyperthyroidism.

Drugs to hypothyroidism: in this case, synthetic thyroid hormones are used to replace the T3 and T4 hormones that are not produced. Among these we have the most commonly used that is Levothyroxine. The side effects are similar to the symptoms of hyperthyroidism (hot flashes, palpitations, insomnia, and nervousness).

Drugs to hyperthyroidism: in the case of hyperthyroidism, the thyroid gland produces its hormones T3 and T4 in excess, exaggerating its physiological effect that causes uncomfortable symptoms for the patient. The drugs used are responsible for blocking the formation of thyroid hormone. Examples of these medications are: methimazole, propylthiouracil, and iodide.

Radioiodine radiations

This therapy is part of nuclear medicine and is used to combat hyperthyroidism. It involves swallowing a small dose of this substance, which is absorbed into the bloodstream and destroys thyroid cells. It is also very effective against thyroid cancer. Side effects associated with this therapy include nausea, vomiting, dry mouth, swelling in the neck, pain in the salivary glands and changes in taste.

Surgery and goiter

When having goiter, an alternative is surgery that removes the thyroid gland totally or partially. It is a procedure that is performed in a maximum of four hours and takes place through an incision above the collarbone. In many cases a catheter is placed to drain blood and fluids. This surgery is recommended in case of excessively large goiter, which affects functions such as breathing and feeding.

Among the side effects and complications arising from surgery we find infections or bruises on the skin, long-term alteration of the voice, respiratory complications due to poor praxis and lower calcium in the blood.

Management after surgery, radioiodine and cancer

After surgery, domestic care is based on excellent wound hygiene and good nutrition. You must take three meals a day based on soft foods and it is essential to be well hydrated.

Once radioactive iodine was applied, the precautions that follow are based on not transmitting iodine radiation to other people. The first thing to keep in mind is not being in contact with young children or pregnant women.
It is ideal to have a separate bathroom or, if it is not possible, the chain must be thrown twice after each use of the toilet. It is better to use disposable cutlery or have cutlery only for the patient, which should be washed separately from others. Also it's advisable to drink a lot of water.

For life after thyroid cancer is necessary to be very attentive to the appearance of symptoms once the treatment is completed; in this case you should talk immediately with your doctor. Food and exercise will be recommended by the physician, and these should be strictly followed according to their indications.

Chapter 7

Physical activity

Resting vs. physical exercise

Although thyroid problems are treated with medication, regular physical exercise has been shown to have very positive effects on people with hypothyroidism. When practicing of physical exercise regularly it increases the levels of T3 and T4.

However, at some points of the treatment you need to rest, for example, after having a thyroid surgery. You must rest at least for three weeks. Otherwise, recovery can be unnecessarily prolonged or have setbacks.

Complications and associated diseases

The problems associated with exercise in the case of these diseases are linked to overweight, fatigue, brittle bones and heart problems. Therefore, if the exercise is not controlled, we are exposed to:

- Hot flushes
- Dizziness
- Joint injuries

- Fracture

Benefits from combined cardio/resistance/elasticity and flexibility routines

When we talk about physical exercise, we do not only refer to weightlifting or walking on the treadmill. Physical exercise should be holistically encompassed. Therefore, the routine is precisely what we must escape from when we seek true benefits.

It is common to get used to an instructor and, much worse, a single type of class that this professional teaches. However, practicing a single mode of exercise takes away the effectiveness of what we are doing.

So the first recommendation to follow is to practice as many classes as possible. On the other hand, the combination of cardio, resistance, elasticity and flexibility, will allow us to burn fat, tone the muscles and obtain the widest possible range of motion. Therefore, we will be protecting our joints and making the exercise more effective every day.

Chapter 8

Dietary measures

There are specific dietary measures for people with hyperthyroidism and with hypothyroidism. These are the following:

Dietary measures for hypothyroidism

You should avoid:

- **Energy bars**
- **Sugars**
- **Processed carbohydrates**
- **Soy products**
- **Coffee**
- **Food genetically modified**
- **Gluten**

It's advisable to eat:

- **Vegetables without starchy**
- **Healthy fats (unsaturated and poly-unsaturated)**
- **Proteins**
- **Vitamins and minerals**

Dietary measures for hyperthyroidism

You should avoid:

- **Algae**
- **Transgenic fats**
- **Dairy products**
- **Soy**
- **Corn**
- **Chemical additives**
- **Caffeine**
- **Sugar**
- **Refined carbohydrates**

You can eat:

- **Almonds**
- **Turnips**
- **Parsley**
- **Flax seeds**
- **Melissa tea**
- **Ajuga herb**

Rich iodine diet

To prevent goiter it is important to have this kind of diet. The foods you should eat are the following:

- Cod
- Blueberries

- Mackerel
- Tuna
- Mussels
- Bean
- Prawns
- Strawberries
- Potatoes
- Cheese
- Salmon
- Cashew nuts
- Broccoli
- Oysters
- Oat
- Peneaut

Low iodine diet

It is indicated when there is an excess of iodine in your body. Therefore, you should avoid the foods detailed above. However, this is all that you are allowed to:

- Egg white
- River fish
- Spices: cinnamon, oregano, pepper
- Potatoes
- Apple
- Blackberries
- Pineapple

- Legumes
- Diet cereals
- Root vegetables
- Homemade bread

Normal iodine diet

It is unspecific, there is no medical indication to increase or reduce the intake of iodine, so you are may consume daily:

- Under 14 years old: 90 mgr/day
- 15 years and more: 150 mgr/day

Gluten intolerance

You can be celiac, which is detected by a blood test, or you can have gluten intolerance. This last is a condition that manifests with vomiting and diarrhea especially in kids, while in adults the symptoms become blurred and there is nothing clear. There is no way to accurately detect that a person is gluten intolerant.

Since the only way to avoid the symptoms of this chronic disease is not to consume gluten, it is convenient that if digestive problems are generated, however minimal, try to eliminate this protein from the diet.

The following ingredients content it and so that should be avoided:

- **Wheat**
- **Oat**
- **Barley**
- **Rye**

Hypothyroidism is a disease strongly related to this pathology.

Lactose intolerance

In this disease the intestine is not able to digest the sugar present in milk (lactose). It is does not cause damage, but has very annoying symptoms, such as colic, diarrhea, nausea and abdominal swelling.

Each person lives it in a different way, so the restriction of food with lactose can be total or partial. We need to know what we should not eat, for example, dairy products. In this diet, the person needs to ingest calcium and vitamin D from other foods. Among them we recommend:

- Citric
- Walnuts
- Omelet

- Plantains
- Tomatoes
- Lettuce
- Carrots
- Olive oil
- Pear
- Pineapple
- Diet bread
- Jams
- Spinach
- Salmon
- Chia seeds
- Free lactose yogurt
- Big wave
- Peneaut butter
- Apple

Most recommended recipes

The most recommended recipes are those that keep the properties and nutrients of the food. Therefore, the following recommendations should be consider:

- Squeeze the citrus at the time
- Grind the seeds at the time of consumption
- Steam cooking

- When it boils, try not to throw water, but it is absorbed
- Do not overcooked Baked foods
- Do not burn Grilled foods
- Cooked vegetables: people with hypothyroidism should not eat raw vegetables, since they give off a toxic substance that prevents iodine absorption.
- Fermented vegetables: recipes such as sauerkraut can be consumed by people with hypothyroidism, since while fermenting, vegetables eliminate the toxic component that prevents iodine from being absorbed.

Menu examples

This is a good menu example for people with hypothyroidism

Breakfast

- 1 cup of yogurt
- ½ cup of big wave
- 3 strawberries

Lunch

- 1 Quesadilla of varied cheeses (such as cheddar), carrot and broccoli
- 1 cup of cocoa mousse

Snack

- 1 slice of diet plantain bread
- 1 cup of liquid yogurt

Dinner

- Mushrooms omelet with cheese
- ½ portion of mussels

Attractive and healthy culinary recipes

Spinach with salad and mango fruit

- Spinach
- Arugula leaves
- 1 Mango fruit
- Olive oil
- 10 walnuts

Wash spinach well and remove the central rib and cut into strips. Add the diced mango, thick chopped walnuts, cut arugula leaves and bathe them with a drizzle of olive oil.

Cucumber and avocado gazpacho

- 2 cucumbers
- 1 Avocado
- 1 Spoon flax seeds
- ½ Liter of water

Peel the fruits and cut them into pieces. Place them in the blender with the rest of the ingredients. Blend until a smooth paste. You can serve it with parsley, basil or chopped walnuts on top.

Chapter 9

Vitamins and minerals

Thyroid gland can get ill due to multiple causes. There is nothing that guarantees 100% that it will keep it running optimally. However, there are certain nutrients that, improve the functions of thyroid gland, and when our diet is lack of them it is more likely to fail. These nutrients are:

Iodine

When the amount of iodine ingested is not enough, the thyroid is not able of producing hormones. We can find iodine in seafood, dairy, sea fish, fruits and vegetables.

Zinc

If this mineral is missing, T3, a hormone that produces the thyroid, cannot reach the DNA. On the other hand, this mineral is important to prostatic functioning, for reproductive organs, the liver and for healing. We find it in pecan nuts, in algae, in dark chocolate, in oysters, in pumpkin seeds, in eggs and in legumes.

Selenium

This mineral helps in the reaction to transform T4 into T3, which is the active thyroid hormone itself. The main problem with this mineral is that, since it comes from food and many countries do not have it as part of their soil, it is essential to take it as a capsule supplement. The foods that have it, as long as the country's soil possesses it, are Brazil nuts, garlic, eggs, blue fish, shellfish, sunflower and mustard seeds, whole grain wheat bread and brown rice.

Iron

It must be present for the thyroid gland to synthesize hormones. We find iron in legumes, so it is very important not to strain the water after cooking. Therefore, it is necessary to use the amount of water necessary, but not more, for cooking according to the amount of legumes. This is because most of the iron remains in the water in which they are cooked. Other foods with iron are milk with iron, shellfish and spinach.

Vitamin A

This is kind of a bridge between thyroid hormone and cellular DNA, where the hormone acts. Without vitamin A, the cells cannot take advantage of thyroid hormones. We find it in the egg yolk, in the sweet potatoes, in the apricots, in the peach, in the melon, in the pumpkin, in the mango and in the papaya.

Chapter 10

Medicinal plants

Beneficial medicinal plants

Some plants are beneficial as a treatment for thyroid gland diseases. It is good to know about so as to prepare a tea or an infusion eventually.

Plants to strengthen immune system

- **Echinacea:** it strengthens the immune system and protects you against viruses and bacteria. It also relieves pain and kills infections.

- **Astragalus Chinese:** it gives balance to nervous system, increases immunity, promotes a good mood and restores vitality.

- **Ginger:** it has excellent digestive function, it is anti-inflammatory, antiseptic and strengthens the immune system.

- **Turmeric:** this is an antioxidant, so it reverses the effect of free radicals and protects cells; it is anti-cancer and strengthens the immune system.

Plants that regulate iodine

- **Evening primrose oil:** it stops hair loss and regulates iodine.

- **Nettle:** this has high iodine content, so it helps to provide it when it is missing.
- **Licorice:** not only regulates iodine, but also stimulates the production of T4 and T3.

- **Flaxseed:** it keeps iodine levels stable and improves thyroid functions.

Harmful plants

In nature, not all plants are safe. There are some which can be really harmful to health. In this case we will talk about those that cause disturbances in the thyroid gland functions (goitrogenic and carcinogenic).

Goitrogenic plants

Goitrogenic plants are those that makes difficult to absorb iodine. Sometimes these plants have a substance which interferes with the iodine in the intestine so the mineral cannot be absorbed. They cannot be consumed by people with hypothyroidism. Some examples of these are cabbage and yucca.

Carcinogenic plants

- **Crotonflavens tea (Euphorbiaceae)**

It was discovered that people from Curacao, which use to drink this tea, has a risk of esophageal cancer 11% higher than the rest of the world.

Chapter 11

Natural supplements

There are some natural supplements commercialized by companies such as Life, which are recommended for people with thyroid gland diseases. These are:

Purely Holistic: it helps thyroid gland to keep their functions through the regulation of the iodine levels. Also, it's good to blood pressure.

Vita Source Labs: its main ingredient is selenium, which produces selenoprotein. This is a very important nutrient for cells function.

Adrenal Work: it is good to control anxiety and stress. Restores the function of adrenal glands and keep your body with energy.

Body Thyroid Support: it has magnesium and cayenne pepper, which accelerates and regulates the metabolism. It's useful to lose weight.

Pure Encapsulations: restores the cells function because of the content of vitamins and minerals that it has.

Now Thyroid Energy: it has iodine and tyrosine, so helps in the production of thyroid hormones. Also contents zinc, copper and selenium, minerals which are important to thyroid function.

Chapter 12

Alternative therapies

These are a group of techniques which are focused on struggling with diseases and pathologies through the activation of some special points in the body. These consider traditional medicine as too invasive and with too many side effects that can be avoided with these techniques.

Stress control

- **Have more social life:** having a lot of friends is good to improve your social life. It helps you to reduce stress, and takes you away from troubles for a while.

- **Increase your good sense of humor:** you need to look for things that make you happy and make you laugh. Those things are good to improve your feelings and health.

- **Sport and physical activity:** practicing sport or physical activity is good for your mood because it releases some hormones in the body that make you feel more comfortable. You can look for yoga, dancing or gymnastic.

Avoid fasting

Though fasting is a recommended technique to eliminate and detoxify your body, it has a lot of side effects which can be worse. When having hyperthyroidism, fasting is banned. Its side effects are:

- Muscle cramps
- Acute back pain
- Fluid retention
- Hypoglycemia
- Headaches
- Sleep disturbance
- Electrolyte imbalance

Therapies against sadness

- **It is okay be sad sometimes**
- **Talk about your feelings**
- **Avoid working too much**
- **Look for a hobby**
- **Practice resilience** (going with positive feelings through difficult situations in life)

Topic IV

Polycystic Ovary Syndrome

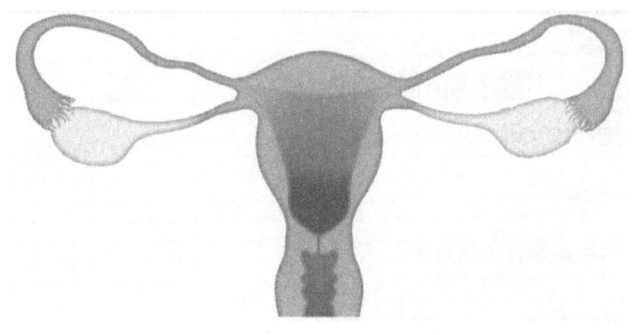

Chapter 1

Concept

Polycystic ovarian syndrome (PCOS) is a very common hormonal disorder among women in reproductive age. Due to the presence of high levels of androgens (male hormones), the ovaries fail to successfully release mature ovules. This causes the mature ovule to be encapsulated within a sphere of fluid within the ovary, although it does not always occur in this way.

When we talk about male hormones in a woman, we might wonder if this is something abnormal, but it isn't at all. The ovaries produce estrogen, progesterone and androgens, and these are male hormones that must be present in women but in low levels. The problem occurs when the amount that is produced is greater than normal.

Adrenal glands also produce androgens, which have the function of regulating the menstrual cycle and ovulation. However, the excess of these hormones has the opposite effect: instead of triggering the release of ovules, it retains inside the ovary. This produces, in some cases, the enlargement of the ovaries.

Polycystic ovary syndrome cam be suspected when the girl or woman start suffering from a lot of annoying symptoms, which leads to diagnosis and treatment.

We must consider that one or several of its symptoms, is not a specific sign of this disease, because it is a physical examination carried out by a gynecologist or by an endocrinologist which will dictate its diagnosis. Also, some image tests are required.

Chapter 2

Most frequent causes

Among the most frequent causes of PCOS are genetic factors, lifestyle habits and endocrine causes.

Genetic

Daughters of patients with PCOV have a greater risk of having it, and it also occurs when there are relatives with this disease.

Lifestyle

Sedentary is one of the causes that lead to this syndrome. Once the patient starts doing exercises and losing weight, PCOS is easier to treat. Also, having a healthy diet and avoiding sugars and fats can help to manage this disease.

Endocrine causes

There is a discussion about what was first? the polycystic ovary or endocrine disorders. However, both interact in this pathophysiology, so it is very important to look for other endocrine disorders when having a diagnosis of PCOS. The most common endocrine causes are:

Hyperprolactinemia: Prolactin is a hormone produced in the adenohypophysis that regulates breast development and milk production. Its increase above normal levels may be related to menstrual abnormalities and polycystic ovary syndrome.

Hypothyroidism: it occurs because the thyroid gland does not produce enough T4. The patients are more sensitive to cold and any physical activity causes fatigue, among other symptoms, one of them, menstrual disorders.

Cushing's disease: it can occur when adenohypophysis produces excessive adrenocorticotropina hormone. Others symptoms are related to de PCOS.

Gigantism or acromegaly: these are diseases that cause excessive limb growth. Gigantism occurs before the epiphysis is closed, while once it is closed, the disease that occurs is acromegaly.

Insulin resistance: it is when insulin is produced normally but the body cannot use it effectively, so blood sugar levels are always high.

Chapter 3

Most common symptoms

While they are annoying and unpleasant, the symptoms help us realize that something strange is happening with our body. Just one symptom does not necessarily say that we have polycystic ovary syndrome. However, when there are several and for no apparent reason, it is advisable to go to the doctor to get a diagnosis. The most common symptoms of polycystic ovary are:

Overweight: there is an increase in weight despite not having changed the diet, and it is very difficult to lose a few grams.

Acne: the sudden appearance of acne, especially in adulthood, may be an indicator of the disease. In the case of adolescence, a worsening in the acne condition can occur.

Oligomenorrhea: it is when the menstrual period occurs infrequently, more that 35 days.

Hirsutism: this is when facial and body hair growth occurs, especially in the back area, around the nipple and in the chest. The hair is excessive and has a male distribution.

Loss hair: hair falls out in much larger quantities than usual.

Chapter 4

Associated disease

Together with PCOS can come some associated diseases, such as:

Abdominal obesity: if the adipose tissue accumulates in the abdomen area, the risks of cardiovascular disease increase. PCOS is associated to obesity and metabolic disorders.

Metabolic Syndrome: this pathology makes fat to accumulate in chest, abdomen, back and hips. It is also related to insulin resistance and, consequently, an increase in insulin production. Therefore, blood sugar accumulates and that increases the presence of adipose tissue.

Fibrocystic breast condition: in this condition there is an alteration in the production of estrogen and progesterone, sex hormones. Symptoms are annoying and painful. There appear some nodules, cysts and even, which can get infected and become abscesses.

Chapter 5

Consequences

Polycystic ovary syndrome is associated with some other pathology such as:

Anovulatory infertility: women with polycystic ovaries usually suffer from infertility related to a failure of the hypothalamus. A natural way to treat this disease is to avoid the intake of saturated animal fats and eat more fruits and vegetables.

Diabetes: it is due to the insulin resistance generated by PCOS, which is the prelude to diabetes. The intake of flax seed is recommended, because it decreases the presence of androgens and helps in their transport through bloodstream, which protects the body from the effects of this disease.

Ischemic heart disease: when unattended or poorly treated PCOS, the possibility of cardiovascular diseases increases because there are high lipid levels in blood. This coronary heart disease is characterized by arteriosclerosis in the arteries of the heart, which can lead to a heart attack. Eating fruits and vegetables, reducing alcohol, and doing physical exercise are the best ways to prevent the ischemic heart disease.

Uterine cancer: women who suffer PCOS have higher risks of developing endometrial cancer.

Gluten intolerance: this is very common when having PCOS, and can be controlled by dietary measures.

Chapter 6

Treatments

Drugs used to treat PCOS

To treat PCOS doctors focus on the conditions of the patient and her wishes of having kids. Combinations of non-pharmacological measures, such as diet and exercise, are usually used, together with medications that will act on the different causes that lead to PCOS. Hormonal contraceptives and medications for insulin resistance can be used.

The first step of the treatment will be a period of 3 to 6 months under a diet, combined with aerobic exercise to lose weight. In a second stage drugs are introduced. **Insulin-sensitizing medications** such as **Metformin** are used to improve the hormonal and metabolic alterations of PCOS.

Hormonal contraceptives are estrogen and progestogen preparations that regulate the hormonal alterations of the female cycle in PCOS; contraceptives that have an antiandrogenic effect are generally used, that is, they block the action of masculinizing hormones, which is increased in PCOS. This improves symptoms such as hirsutism and loss hair. Some of these medications are:

Cyproterone Acetate, Chlormadinone Acetate, Dinogest, and Drospirenone.

For women who wish to have babies, a drug called **Clomiphene** can be used alone or in combination with **metformin**; its function is to stimulate ovulation. These patients may also need specialized fertilization.

Some side effects of the medication are: alterations of the menstrual cycle and alterations of the metabolism, gastrointestinal symptoms such as nausea, vomiting, diarrhea, hypotension and dizziness

In vitro Fertilization

It's in an alternative for infertility due to PCOS. The cells used may be from the same woman who is going to be a mother or a donor. The same goes for sperm. Another option is the surrogate mother, who lends the womb for pregnancy.

The complication in assisted fertilization is multiple pregnancy. But it can also be prevented by placing a smaller amount of embryos to the future mother.

Ovary Surgery

There are two types of preventive ovarian surgeries. One of them is laparoscopy and the other is abdominal.

Laparoscopic surgery is performed under local anesthesia and the ovaries are removed through an incision in the navel that allows the entry of a tube. It lasts around an hour and a half. Abdominal removal is done under general anesthesia, the bikini cut is performed to carry it out and can last two hours.

The advantages offered by these surgeries is removing the problems related to polycystic ovaries. The disadvantages can include infections, hemorrhages, intestinal obstruction, scar tissue formation and possible injuries to internal organs. Of course, lifelong infertility is the most direct consequence.

Chapter 7

Physical activity

Practicing physical exercise is very important in PCOS, because it helps to control body weight, which and also physical exercise improves reproductive function.

Benefits from cardio/resistance/elasticity and flexibility combined routines

It is recommended to do at least two and a half hours of weekly aerobic physical exercise. The intensity will vary as the body becomes more trained and develops its lung capacity to the fullest. The recommendation is to do it as intensely as possible.

Time should be divided into sessions of a minimum of thirty minutes and a maximum of forty-five.

Water gymnastics is especially recommended for these women, as well as Zumba, since it helps improve mood.

At least twice a week, a resistance routine should be performed covering all muscle groups. Sessions should last one hour. When muscle is developed, more calories are burned.

Finally, elasticity and flexibility will help to improve the exercise of bodybuilding, because avoid pain and cramps, so exercise will be more effective every day. It is necessary to stretch each muscle worked for a minimum of twenty seconds after the sessions of bodybuilding and aerobics, as well as perform physical activities specially designed to gain flexibility, such as ballet, yoga, Pilates and stretching

Chapter 8

Dietary measures

Eating a healthy diet is the key to avoid associated diseases and other consequences of PCOS. Because this syndrome causes hyperglycemia can lead to diabetes and overweight. However, by eating a healthy diet both can be prevented.

Carbohydrates are the axis around which everything must circulate. We cannot forget them, even knowing that they are responsible for raising blood sugar. That is why we must know which ones to choose. Not all carbohydrates are the same, but some have more impact in blood sugar. It is necessary to learn to choose in the right way.

The most suitable carbohydrates for women suffering from PCOS are:

- **Fresh fruits**
- **Fresh vegetables**
- **Rich fiber cereals** (5gr of fiber per portion)
- **Yogurt sugar free**

The following foods should be avoided:

- **Starchy vegetables**
- **Refined carbohydrates and cereals** (flour, rice)
- **Cookies, cakes**

Low calorie diet

This diet is an option to keep weight within normal parameters. However, getting involved in such a diet requires that we know our body a lot.

First, the definition of a low calorie diet is to eat few calories than what we spend. It sounds simple, but it is not. To avoid having a deficit diet, we must find out how many calories our body spends at baseline, and then add calories that we spend according to the exercise we do.

The basal metabolic expenditure depends on a number of factors, such as height, age and the speed of our metabolism, so we can realize following this diet is not that easy. A way to know it is through the Harris – Benedict equation:

Man: 66,473 + (13,751 x weight kg) + (5,0033 x height cm) – (6,7550 x age)

Woman: 655,1 + (9,463 x weight kg) + (1,8 x height cm) – (4,6756 x age)

To this result you need to add the calories you expend while doing exercise.

To avoid the rebound effect of these diets is not to lower the calories we consume to less than 300 of those we spend.

On the other hand, if we have to talk about rebound effect, we are not in proper eating plan. So it is better to have a healthy diet rather than going on diets that lead us to lose weight drastically, but are not sustainable over time.

Diet to treat acne

Acne is another side effect of PCOS. In this case, diet should be free of saturated fats and replaced by omega 3 fats. For example, both butter and chocolate are contraindicated. Instead, here is a list of highly recommended foods to prevent acne:

- Tuna
- Salmon
- Chia seeds
- Nuts
- Green vegetables
- Broccoli
- Carrots
- Yogurt
- Water
- Avocado
- Garlic

- Turmeric

Diet to treat hyperandrogenism

When suffering from hyperandrogenism, you should reduce testosterone levels, and diet can help on it. The foods recommended are:

- Almonds
- Walnuts
- Linseed flour
- Flax seeds
- Licorice
- Peppermint
- Mint
- Tuna
- Salmon
- Herring
- Sardines
- Onion

What can be food according to glycemic index

Because hyperglycemia is a serious problem for women with PCOS, it is better to choose foods that have a low GI (glycemic index), and do not cause blood sugar levels to rise. Examples of these foods are:

- **Legumes**

- **Vegetable**
- **Diet bread**
- **Diet rice**

Most recommended recipes

They way of cooking also affects the glycemic index in foods. Some good preparations are:

- Nuts
- Fresh fruits
- Eat fruits rather than just drinking juice
- Eat baked potatoes instead of mash potatoes
- Choose diet bread
- Don't cook foods too much

If we are going to choose one food with a high glycemic index, we must combine it with other which low glycemic index.

Menu examples

These are some recommended recipes for patients with PCOS:

Breakfast: two slides of diet bread with peanut butter and a glass of cocoa milk.

Lunch: ravioli with fresh tomato sauce and as a dessert a fruit.

Snack: two rice cookies with berries jams without sugar and a cup of natural yogurt.

Dinner: diet rice with tuna and peppers. The dessert can be vanilla cream.

Attractive and healthy culinary recipes

Broccoli au gratin with cheddar cheese and egg

Ingredients

- ½ Kg of broccoli
- ¼ Litter of béchamel sauce
- 2 eggs
- 200gr cheddar cheese
- Cayena pepper
- Turmeric

First, boil the broccoli and the eggs. Then prepare the béchamel sauce and add a quarter liter of milk. Put the broccoli in a baking dish, put the sliced eggs on top, cover them with the béchamel sauce and put the grated cheddar cheese on top.

The oven should be preheated at 180° C, put the dish and cook 15 minutes until gratin. Then serve hot.

Salmon and Walnut salad

Ingredients

- 1 slice of smoked salmon
- 1 peeled tomato
- Arugula leaves
- Lettuce leaves
- 10 walnuts
- Olive oil

Peel the tomato without scalding it, cut the arugula leaves and lettuce into strips and cut the nuts in half. Arrange everything in a bowl and sprinkle with olive oil. Serve cold or natural.

Chapter 9

Vitamins and minerals

Some essential nutrients prevent and help in the management of PCOS. The following are those you should keep in your diet:

Vitamins

- Vitamin A
- Vitamin C
- Vitamin D
- Inositol (B complex vitamin)

Minerals

- Chrome
- Zinc

Foods rich in vitamin A

- Dairy products
- Eggs
- Mango
- Cabbage
- Spinach

- Sweet potatoes
- Broccoli
- Carrots
- Legumes
- Fish
- Seafood

Food rich in vitamin C

- Citrus
- Pineapple
- Papaya
- Mango
- Fruit melon
- Watermelon
- Red and green peppers
- Cidrayotec
- Tomato
- Potatoes
- Sweet potatoes

Food rich in vitamin D

- Mushrooms
- Salmon
- Tuna
- Cheese
- Eggs

Food rich in Inositol

- Plantains
- Cereals with bran
- Integral rice
- Oat
- Beans
- Citrus
- Wheat germ
- Grapes and plums

Food rich in chrome

- Onion
- Diet cereals
- Tomato
- Fruits

Food rich in zinc

- Eggs
- Oysters
- Clams
- Hazelnuts
- Almonds
- Cascaded
- Cheese
- Oat

Chapter 10

Medicinal plants

Beneficial medicinal plants

In nature are the ingredients that help regulate our metabolism and endocrine system. When having PCOS, we need to find plants that reduce testosterone, regulate the menstrual cycle, enhance fertility and improve insulin resistance.

Plants to reduce testosterone

- Mint
- Peppermint
- Sage
- Ruda cabruna
- Licorice

Plants to treat menstrual disorders

- Ginger
- Verbena
- Chamomile
- Sage
- Rosemary

Plants to treat infertility

- Nettle
- Dandelion
- Wild oats
- Wild yam
- Dong quai
- Chaste berry
- Green tea

Plants to improve insulin resistance

- Passionflower
- Chamomile
- Orange blossom
- Balm
- Dandelion
- Artichoke
- Pennyroyal
- Green anise

Chapter 11

Natural supplements

Companies as Life, have been working on researching how to gather the best natural supplements and encapsulate them so you can deal with the symptoms of polycystic ovaries. The most used supplements are:

- **My Ova Myo-plus:** its myoinositol helps in mood balance, reduces blood glucose levels, and regulates the menstrual cycle. In turn, it restores the correct hormonal dynamics and makes the ovaries function properly.
- **PCOS Capsules:** it regulates the menstrual cycle, reduces facial and body hair when it is excessive due to excess testosterone and prevents diabetes. It is made up of more than 10 essential vitamins and minerals. After six weeks of consuming it daily, the mood changes completely.
- **Soria Natural Melatonin:** Melatonin is a hormone that is secreted during sleep and that regulates ovulation. This can repair the oxidative damage within the ovule, improves progesterone levels and the quality of the receptors
- **Simply supplement folic acid:** this nutrient prevents and slows down the oxidation of the ovules, so it is very beneficial to improve fertility.

Chapter 12

Alternative therapies

Apart from having the traditional medicinal options, we also have new therapies to treat PCPS and its consequences, in the nature.

To treat acne

- **Phytotherapy:** it uses plants and herbs to treat many diseases.

- **Mesotherapy:** it consists in the application of subcutaneous micro-injections, which contain vitamins, minerals and amino acids that fight the causes of acne.

- **Homeopathy:** in this practice are used some natural products, diets and other therapies that can treat acne in a natural way.

To treat hirsutism

- **Herbs:** it is good to prepare a tea with a teaspoon of herb for every quarter liter of water. The indicated herbs are: black cohosh, saw palmetto, chaste tree and mint tea.

- **Glycerin:** glycerin extract is good to threat hirsutism.

- **Acupuncture:** needles are placed at strategic points of the body to inhibit hair growth.

To treat infertility

- **Acupuncture**
- **Reflexology**
- **Hypnosis**
- **Homeopathy**

To control weight

- **Acupuncture:** when the membrane of the skin breaks, the production of endorphins is triggered, so that appetite is reduced immediately.
- **Acupressure:** pressure in different parts of the body also reduces the sensation of hunger, especially that produced merely by anxiety.
- **Hypnosis:** in this technique you are taken to project a new image of you, the one you would like to see every day in the mirror. Therefore, when you leave the trance, you are ready to do whatever it takes to get it
- **Reflexology:** there are specific areas of the sole of the foot are pressed to stimulate the organs responsible for suppressing appetite.

Topic V

Menopause and Andropause

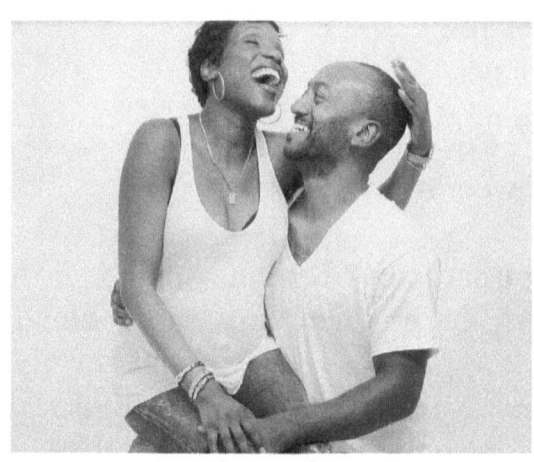

Chapter 1

Concept

Menopause and Andropause take place, in women and men, at middle age. These are permanent and irreversible changes which happen because of age and their result is the cessation of reproductive function in women and the decrease in sexual function in men.

This period covers many years, since it begins with pre-menopause, it is extended by menopause itself and continues until the end of post menopause, in case of women.

The changes are biological, psychological, emotional and social.

Types

Andropause: in men it happens around fifty years old. The body produces less testosterone and the man experiences symptoms very similar to those manifested in menopause in women, such as decrease in libido, lower intellectual performance and decreased vitality.

Menopause: this is a period of life in women where lots of changes occur, it goes from pre-menopause to post menopause. It can start around fifty years old or before.

Specifically, menopause is a term used to refer to the last menstruation that a woman had. Menopause starts because of ovaries stop producing female hormones. Therefore, menopause ends the reproductive capacity of women. As estrogens and progesterone are not present, some organs that need them begin to deteriorate. That is why it is recommended to replace them with synthetic hormones in some cases.

Early menopause: it occurs between forty-one and forty-seven years old. Early menopause does not necessarily have health consequences, as it is within the expected age range.

Premature menopause: It happens before forty years old. The cause is the same that in the current menopausal, and also can occur early when the woman has gone through an ovary extirpation surgery or after chemotherapy or radiotherapy. Genetics can also influence. Usually this isn't a problem, sometime it is necessary to get some exams to detect the cause. It is important to remember that contraceptive methods must be used as long as the doctor determines that there is no possibility of egg release.

Chapter 2

Most frequent causes

Some factors which can have influence in menopause and andropause can be genetic factors, lifestyle habits and endocrine causes.

Genetic

It is more common in menopause. If there is someone in family which had premature or early menopause with too many symptoms that required treatment, the women have more risk.

Lifestyle habits

Smoking is related to menopause and andropause early in life. In this case the person is likely to suffer from more intense symptoms.

Endocrine Causes

Endocrine diseases are related to early menopause/andropause because both are influenced by hormones. The diseases more frequents are:

- **Insulin resistance**

- **Polycystic ovary syndrome**

- **Hypothyroidism**
- **Cushing's disease**
- **Hypogonadism**
- **Gigantism or acromegaly**

Other medical causes

Some treatments are related to early onset of menopause/andropause symptoms, such as:

Chemotherapy or radiotherapy: Treatments against cancer may damage the structure of the ovary, affecting its hormonal production.

Surgery to remove uterus: Also known as hysterectomy, in this surgery often ovaries al also removed.

Surgery to remove ovaries: the effect is immediate, as the hormonal level drops abruptly with this operation. The menstruation stops and the menopause starts.

Chapter 3

Most common symptoms

Men and women are different, and their way of living this period is very different. Each one of them suffers symptoms that are experienced differently, though some may be similar too.

Common symptoms in men

- Demotivation
- Lack of energy
- Loss of muscle strength
- Drowsiness
- Hair loss

Common symptoms in women
- Menstrual disorders
- Hot flushes
- Insomnia
- Fatigue
- Depression
- Irritability

It is possible for men to experience strong anguish and desire to cry inexplicably, but these psychological symptoms are more common in women.

Chapter 4

Associated diseases

Some diseases that can come together with menopause and andropause are:

Obesity: The metabolism slows down men and women become overweight. This is due to the decrease in estrogen and the lower energy wear associated with age.
High blood pressure: this is related to the increase in body mass, which makes the pressure to pump blood to the heart greater.
Dyslipidemia: the decrease in estrogen affects the cleaning of blood from lipids, so any fatty food stays in the body causing damage.
Diabetes: Estrogens have the function of keeping the blood and arteries clean to control sugar and lipid levels. When decreasing, insulin resistance may occur and lead to diabetes.
Hypothyroidism: due to hormonal changes, the thyroid begins to fail in its functions.
Emotional disorders: hormonal changes affect psychology. It is common to go from laughter to crying without reason. If these symptoms are not treated, they could lead to depression or anxiety.

Chapter 5

Consequences

Osteoporosis: During this period is when more bone mass is lost. This leads to risks of fractures. However, there are natural ways to reverse this process and lead a completely healthy life. First, it is recommended to practice low impact exercises, such as some kinds of gymnastics. This makes the muscle grow, so it protects and regenerates bone mass. To get more calcium there are vegetables that contain even more than dairy products, for example of this is parsley. Finally, since coffee is a very potent decalcifying agent, it is recommended to avoid it.

Ischemic heart disease: the deterioration and the possible obstruction of the coronary arteries can be treated with natural methods. An aerobic routine and avoiding sedentary lifestyle is the first step. After two months of starting an exercise program, you will begin to notice the improvements.

Infertility: this is part of the natural process of aging; infertility is total for women, while men may have a sexual impairment.

Sexual impairment: Loss of potency and sexual desire associated with the climacteric can be restored through foods that raise libido and allow better blood supply to the male genitals. Among them we find onion, seafood and ginger.

Depression: Hormonal changes affect both female and male psychology. Fortunately, there are measures that can be taken to manage these feelings, sadness and depression. Practicing a sport that motivates us, making new friends and staying in close to things or people we like are three basic measures to start this new stage of life.

Chapter 6

Treatments

Medications

Hormonal replacement therapy for Andropause:

In the andropause, the main symptoms arise from the decrease in testosterone levels, which is the male hormone par excellence. When this hormone is low, the symptoms are complaints about sexual function. The hormone replacement therapy in this case is based on administering testosterone or its analogues to restore these levels and recover male sexual function. The following preparations are currently available:

- **Testosterone esters** (ester testosterone enanthate): this comes in an oily preparation for intramuscular administration every 21 days as it is slowly absorbed.
- **Testosterone undecanoate**: it is also one of the testosterone esters but it is administered orally several times a day because its metabolism is rapid. There are slower presentations available in injections.
- **Transdermal testosterone:** This type of testosterone is administered directly to the skin in gels or patches. Gels are preferred to apply to the

armpits, shoulders, and abdomen, early in the morning and you should wait at least 6 hours to wet the area. It is a treatment that allows constant release of testosterone from the skin to the blood, recommended in patients over 40 years.

Testosterone should be administered with caution, since its adverse effects include heart problems and prostate pathologies.

Hormonal replacement for Menopause:

The treatment of menopause will depend on how the patient is living this experience. If the symptoms are not bothersome or harm your quality of life, the therapy is based on non-pharmacological measures such as: promote a healthy diet free of fats and condiments, perform aerobic physical exercise such as gymnastics or cycling on a regular basis, avoid habits healthy as smoking or drinking alcohol and coffee in excess, control other diseases that suffer from hypertension, perform regular tests for osteoporosis and breast cancer, and maintain a positive attitude to life.

However, if the symptoms are bothersome for the patients, then a hormone replacement therapy is recommended. This should start with the minimum effective dose and is aimed at the treatment of vasomotor symptoms (hot flashes) and urogenital (vaginitis, itching, inflammation) due to estrogen deficiency

Estrogen therapy is recommended in women before age 60, as well as for short periods of time, as it is associated with certain risks such as increased incidence of breast and endometrial cancer.

The following combinations are use:

- **Estrogens (alone)**: this decreases the symptoms of pain, hot flashes, hot flashes, itching and vaginal infections, and improves osteoporosis.
- **Estrogens and progestogens**: they have the same estrogenic effects already described. Combined progestogens are used when the woman has not been hysterectomized, to counteract the effects of estrogen in excess.
- **Tibolona**: this is a medication that enters the body is transformed into estrogen, progestogen and androgenic derivatives. It is used to treat symptoms of estrogen deficiency in menopause, such as sweating, hot flashes, changes in libido and mood.

Among the possible side effects we can find visual disturbances, itching, vomiting, edema, weight gain, increased cardiovascular risk, dyslipidemia and increased risk of venous obstruction (thrombosis).

Surgeries

Lately there has been a strong advent of surgeries related to counteracting the visible effects of menopause. We highlight the following:

Aesthetics: the body stops producing collagen, so the skin is refined and the sagging effect occurs. To reverse it, there are facial and neck rejuvenation surgeries. Through lifting or injection techniques, the lush appearance is returned to the face.

Hair implants: men lose a lot of hair; they turn out to be the most numerous clients of this treatment. It consists of implanting hair from populated areas of the head to those that have lost hair. Local anesthesia is used to perform. Some risks in this surgery are infections and the aggravation of the problem of baldness.

Genitals: in this surgery you have both, an aesthetic and functional purpose. While they improve the visible appearance of the genitals, they also solve problems such as urinary incontinence. They help improve self-esteem because provide a youthful look in the area. Men can also perform multiple genital cosmetic surgeries, which include penis enlargement and thickening, as well as scrotal lifting. The benefit is a better sexual function, while the risks could be just the opposite: loss of genital sensation, both in men and women, due to nerve damage in the area.

Chapter 7

Physical activity

Each stage of life has its good things and its challenges. The good news is that physical exercise can come with us to help. We just have to be careful when practicing it because menopause/ andropause are periods with some limitations in movements and also problems in health. But it's not about quick it, but about adapting exercise to our new life.

To do an effective exercise, it must be done every day, at least five days a week and for at least forty minutes.

Movement possibilities

The reflexes of the body decreases, so exercise has to be performed at your steps. Some physical activities that you can do are:

- Walking
- Swimming
- Zumba
- Gymnastics
- Cycling
- Weight lifting
- Abdominal exercises

Consequences and related diseases

Menopause is a period where people can have some limitations to do physical exercise. Some problems are:

- Osteoporosis
- Hot flashes
- Insomnia

Thinking of these factors will help us to do a better performance when exercising. First, osteoporosis can cause bone fractures, so we will not choose a skipped aerobic class or a very demanding dance class.

To avoid hot flashes we have to be prepared to exercise with fresh clothes. It is a mistake to belief that the coat makes us lose weight more due to excessive perspiration. This will only lead us to suffocate and have to interrupt the exercise session. Also, you need to drink enough water.

Finally, to avoid insomnia, we must use the exercise in our favor. So it is good to exercise preferably at night and never drink an isotonic drink to hydrate, since it over-excites us, but water will be our best company.

Benefits from cardio/resistance/elasticity and flexibility routines

The exercise should is a holistic practice, so these four activities have to be present. Aerobics should be practiced every day, as well as elasticity and flexibility, while twice a week they are sufficient for resistance, since it involves lifting weights and the body has to recover.

The benefits of physical activity in this period are:

- **Improves mood and self-esteem**
- **Increases agility and cerebellar coordination**
- **Helps to sleep better**
- **Increase lung capacity**
- **Keeps you in normal weight**
- **Improves health**
- **Regulates intestinal peristalsis**
- **Prevents cardiovascular diseases**
- **Prevents osteoporosis**

Chapter 8

Dietary measures

Dietary measures to transit the menopause/andropause will help us prevent diseases, relieve symptoms and improve mood and feelings.

Aphrodisiacs

Aphrodisiacs can return the sexual desire to people who have lost it for physical or emotional reasons. They are very effective, however, we must keep in mind that they do not replace love, but rather exalt it. So without love, little is the effect they will do. The most popular aphrodisiacs are:

- **Andean maca**
- **Ginseng**
- **Coffee**
- **Chocolate**
- **Walnuts**
- **Saffron**
- **Royal jelly**
- **Mint**

Healthy diet

A healthy diet has carbohydrates and calories in the right quantities. This diet needs to have:

- **Carbohydrates**: give energy
- **Proteins:** help to increase muscle mass and heal tissues
- **Unsaturated and poly-unsaturated fats:** transport vitamins and clean our blood from cholesterol.
- **Vitamins and minerals:** helps in the functions of the systems of our body.

Diets to become younger

These diets contain natural antioxidants, which reduce the effect of free radicals. These antioxidants we can find in:
- **Oranges**
- **Mangos**
- **Carrots**
- **Pumpkin**
- **Sweet potatoes**
- **Zucchini**
- **Broccoli**
- **Nuts**
- **Seeds**
- **Spinach**
- **Kale**
- **Green vegetables**
- **Milk**
- **Butter**
- **Eggs**

- **Pink grapefruit**
- **Tomatoes**
- **Watermelon**
- **Cereals**
- **Papaya**
- **Strawberries**
- **Fish**
- **Diet bread**
- **Kiwi**

Natural phytohormones

They are an increasingly accepted alternative for hormone replacement therapy, because it is almost free from risk. Phytohormones are plant hormones that have functions similar to estrogen and testosterone, which are low in the menopause and andropause. We can find them in:

- **Soy**
- **Cereals**
- **Schisandra berries**
- **Green tea**
- **Hops**

Most recommended recipes

The way that we cook food is very important to get nutrients. Some advices for cooking are:

- Choose fruits and vegetables of the season
- When boiling vegetables just put the water needed, so vegetables won't absorbed too much.
- Don't cook too much foods
- Cut or grate the fresh fruits and vegetables just before eating

Menu examples

Breakfast: integral bread with cheese and yogurt.

Lunch: baked fish with potatoes and sweet potatoes.

Snack: cheese cake without sugar and green tea.

Dinner: carrots, broccoli and leeks boiled with tomato sauce.

Attractive and healthy recipes

Mushrooms and zucchini sautéed

- 1 can of mushrooms
- 1 clove garlic
- ½ Onion
- 1 Zucchini
- Olive oil
- Cayena pepper

Cut the garlic into small pieces. Cut the onion into brunoise and diced zucchini. Cut the mushrooms in half. Heat the olive oil in one in a pan. Put the garlic and onion until they barely brown. Add the mushrooms. Finally, add the zucchini and let them cook until they are tender. Turn off the heat and add cayenne pepper.

Watercress, watermelon, melon and avocado salad

- Watercress
- Watermelon
- Melon
- Avocado

Cut all the fruits in cubes without seeds and mixture them. At the end add little lemon juice.

Chapter 9

Vitamins and minerals

There is a certain group of vitamins and minerals which must be present in the diet. They help in the functions of the hormonal system, in the mood and in the prevention of associated diseases in this period.

Vitamins

- Vitamin C
- Vitamin E

Vitamin C helps in the production of estrogens and vitamin E helps to manage hot flashes, excessive sweating, anxiety and insomnia.

Minerals

- **Calcium** – a good quantity recommended is 1.200 – 1.500 mg /day to prevent osteoporosis.

Foods rich in vitamin C

- Persimmon
- Garlic
- Strawberries
- Citrus

- Acerola berries
- Blackcurrant
- Kiwi
- Guava
- Peppers
- Papayas
- Fruit melon
- Amalaki
- Brussels Cabbages

Foods rich in vitamin E

- Green vegetables
- Nuts
- Wheat germ oil, sunflower oil and corn oil
- Seeds

Food rich in calcium

- Dairy products
- Walnuts
- Green vegetables
- Kiwi
- Strawberries
- Cherries
- Brevas
- Figs
- Plums
- Lemon

- Currants
- Papaya
- Blue fishes
- Prawns
- Tofu
- Seeds
- Eggs

Chapter 10

Medicinal plants

Beneficial plants

The plants that are beneficial during menopause/andropause can treat associated diseases, as well as help in the control of our hormonal function, managing symptoms such as hot flashes and sadness.

Plants to lose weight

- Ginseng
- Cayena pepper
- Dandelion
- Black pepper
- Turmeric
- Mustard
- Cinnamon
- Cardamom
- Ginger
- Cumin

Plants that improves hormones

- Dandelion

- Parsley
- Sarsaparilla
- Kelp
- Alfalfa

Plants to treat sadness

- Melissa
- Grass of San Juan
- Ginseng
- Valerian
- Ylang-ylang
- Lavender
- Chamomile
- Poppy
- Estragon
- Sage

Plants to help in sleep disturbances

- Passionflower
- Linden
- Chamomile
- Rosemary
- Mint
- Lemon balm
- Lavender
- Melissa

- Valerian
- Ginseng

Plants to get energy

- Turmeric
- Aloe Vera
- Yerba mate
- Cinnamon and ginseng infusion
- Guarana

Plants to treat hot flashes

- Meadow clover
- Sage
- Cimicifuga
- Hops

Plants to treat menstrual disorders

- Chaste berry
- Evening primrose
- Shepherd's bag
- Cimicifuga
- Chia

Chapter 11

Natural supplements

Some companies, such as Life, create supplements based on natural products. The advantage is that you can get as many nutrients as necessary in a single capsule. With these you do not need to supplement the consumption of these nutrients with other foods.

Whey Protein Evo: it is concentrated whey protein. It gives energy, provides strength and helps to gain muscle mass. Also, it activates the metabolism.
Soy Protein Isolate 2.0: it is vegetable protein from soybeans. It helps muscle development, so it will improve the quality of our physical exercises, allow us to lift more weight, we will be stronger and burn more calories.
Vitamin D3 4000 IU: this is a vitamin D concentrate that comes in pearls. It provides the necessary muscular strength to be able to improve in physical exercises, something vital in menopause.
Omega-3 Ultra: Provides omega 3 fatty acids. It helps the brain function properly, keeps blood cholesterol levels controlled and helps with vision.

Chapter 12

Alternative therapies

If we prefer natural treatments instead of traditional medicine with its procedures and drugs, we can opt for an alternative therapy to help us deal with the symptoms of menopause and andropause.

Behavioral therapies

- **Exposure techniques:** the patient is confronted with the factor that causes fear. It is useful against phobias and anxiety.

- **Systematic desensitization:** it's to treat anxiety by generating behaviors' that prevent its occurrence.

- **Cognitive Restructuring:** the patient's thoughts are modified so that it relieves his/her psychological ailments by moving them away

Stress control

- Laughter therapy
- Aromatherapy
- Infusions
- Meditation

- Yoga
- Cryotherapy (uses cold to stimulate the organism and release serotonin, endorphins and y dopamine)
- Pressotherapy (uses air massage techniques to relax the arms, back, and legs).

Relaxation therapies

- **Breathing**
- **Meditation**
- **Mental journey**
- **Mindfulness**

Anxiety control

- **Aromatherapy**
- **Homeopathy**
- **Laughter therapy**
- **Bach flowers**
- **Phytotherapy**

Depression control

- **Food supplements** (magnesium, vitamin B, Omega 3)
- **Light therapy** (the patient needs to expose to sun)
- **Exercise**

Body image

- Accept your own body
- Make a list of positive aspect about your body
- Expend time with people that love you and respect you
- Be respectful with your body and start by having a healthy diet

Self-esteem

- **Reiki**
- **Chromotherapia**
- **Aromatherapy**
- **Laughter therapy**
- **Hugs therapy**

Occupational therapy

It is about to keep your mind busy so as to avoid thinking of your physical or cognitive conditions. It focuses on make more important your abilities than your weaknesses, and helps you to get in the social world.

References organized by topics and chapters

Topic I. Diabetes

Chapter 1. Definition
- https://www.who.int/es/news-room/fact-sheets/detail/diabetes
- https://kidshealth.org/es/kids/type1-esp.html

Chapter 2. Most frequent causes
- https://www.niddk.nih.gov/health-information/informacion-de-la-salud/diabetes/informacion-general/sintomas-causas
- http://www.diabetes.org/es/informacion-basica-de-la-diabetes/diabetes-gestacional/que-es-la-diabetes-gestacional.html
- http://www.cadime.es/es/noticia.cfm?iid=hiprglucemias-medicamentos#.XQFkk9IzaM8

Chapter 3. Most common symptoms
- https://es.wikipedia.org/wiki/Polidipsia
- https://www.msdmanuals.com/es/professional/trastornos-urogenitales/s%C3%ADntomas-de-los-trastornos-urogenitales/poliuria
- https://www.semiologiaclinica.com/index.php/articlecontainer/motivosdeconsulta/126-polifagia
- https://www.mayoclinic.org/es-es/diseases-conditions/itchy-skin/diagnosis-treatment/drc-20355010
- https://www.niddk.nih.gov/health-information/informacion-de-la-salud/diabetes/informacion-general/sintomas-causas

Chapter 4. Associated diseases
- https://www.mayoclinic.org/es-es/diseases-conditions/yeast-infection/symptoms-causes/syc-20378999
- https://cuidateplus.marca.com/enfermedades/urologicas/balanitis.html
- https://medlineplus.gov/spanish/ency/article/000521.htm
- http://www.diabetes.org/es/vivir-con-diabetes/complicaciones/complicaciones-en-la-piel.html

- http://www.diabetes.org/es/vivir-con-diabetes/tratamiento-y-cuidado/higiene-y-salud-bucal/la-diabetes-y-los-problemas-de-salud-bucal.html

Chapter 5. Consequences, prevention and natural advises for managing
- https://www.mayoclinic.org/es-es/diseases-conditions/peripheral-neuropathy/symptoms-causes/syc-20352061
- https://cuidateplus.marca.com/enfermedades/ginecologicas/disfuncion-sexual-femenina.html
- https://www.niddk.nih.gov/health-information/informacion-de-la-salud/enfermedades-urologicas/disfuncion-erectil/prevencion
- https://cuidateplus.marca.com/enfermedades/urologicas/impotencia-disfuncion-erectil.html
- http://www.kidneyfund.org/en-espanol/enfermedad-de-los-rinones/tipos/enfermedad-de-los-rinones-cronica.html
- http://www.revcardiologia.sld.cu/index.php/revcardiologia/article/view/566/723
- https://fundaciondelcorazon.com/informacion-para-pacientes/enfermedades-cardiovasculares/cardiopatia-isquemica.html
- https://medlineplus.gov/spanish/diabeticfoot.html
- https://medlineplus.gov/spanish/diabeticfoot.html
- http://www.hoy.com.ec/remedios-caseros-para-la-disfuncion-erectil/
- https://www.kidney.org/es/atoz/content/como-afecta-al-cuerpo-la-insuficiencia-renal
- https://holadoctor.com/es/%C3%A1lbum-de-fotos/10-remedios-naturales-para-el-coraz%C3%B3n
- https://mejorconsalud.com/preparar-5-remedios-naturales-las-ulceras-del-pie-diabetico/

Chapter 6. Treatments
- https://es.familydoctor.org/medicamentos-orales-para-la-diabetes/
- http://cirugiavascularactual.blogspot.com/2007/08/pie-diabtico-clasificacin-etapificacin.html
- http://www.diabetes.org/es/vivir-con-diabetes/tratamiento-y-cuidado/transplantes/trasplante-de-pncreas.html

Chapter 7. Physical activity

- https://www.elsevier.es/es-revista-avances-diabetologia-326-articulo-efecto-del-ejercicio-fisico-sobre-S1134323012000385
- https://www.elsevier.es/es-revista-endocrinologia-nutricion-12-articulo-impacto-actividad-fisica-sobre-el-S1575092210000525
- https://www.webconsultas.com/ejercicio-y-deporte/ejercicio-y-enfermedad/ejercicios-recomendados-en-personas-con-diabetes
- https://lopezdoriga.com/vida-y-estilo/diferencia-entre-flexibilidad-y-elasticidad/

Chapter 8. Dietary measures
- http://www.diabetes.org/es/alimentos-y-actividad-fisica/alimentos/que-voy-a-comer/comprension-de-los-carbohidratos/contar-carbohidratos.html
- https://www.dietistasnutricionistas.es/indice-glucemico-la-carga-glucemica/
- https://medlineplus.gov/spanish/ency/patientinstructions/000941.htm
- http://www.diabetes.org/es/alimentos-y-actividad-fisica/alimentos/que-voy-a-comer/consejos-de-comidas/lea-detenidamente-las-etiquetas.html
- https://www.mayoclinic.org/es-es/diseases-conditions/diabetes/in-depth/diabetes-diet/art-20044295
- https://www.fundaciondiabetes.org/general/articulo/169/la-alimentacion-en-la-diabetes-tipo-2--plan-semanal-de-alimentacion
- https://misrecetasparadiabeticos.com/ensaladas-diabeticos/

Chapter 9. Vitamins and minerals
- https://www.niddk.nih.gov/health-information/informacion-de-la-salud/diabetes/informacion-general/nutricion-alimentacion-actividad-fisica/conteo-carbohidratos
- http://diabetesdietas.com/diabetes-minerales-vitaminas-reducen-la-diabetes/

Chapter 10. Medicinal Plants
- https://www.cuerpomente.com/salud-natural/tratamientos/8-plantas-y-suplementos-que-protegen-frente-a-la-diabetes_161
- https://mejorconsalud.com/7-hierbas-te-ayudan-tratar-la-diabetes-tipo-2/
- https://www.saludnutricionbienestar.com/berberina-planta-diabetes/

- https://holadoctor.com/es/%C3%A1lbum-de-fotos/10-hierbas-aliadas-contra-la-diabetes

Chapter 11. Endorsed products for diabetic people
- http://fmdiabetes.org/marcas-avaladas/

Chapter 12. Alternative therapies for managing diabetes
- https://cuidateplus.marca.com/medicamentos/2016/03/03/homeopatia-que-sirve-109987.html
- https://www.vix.com/es/imj/salud/2011/02/17/medicina-alternativa-para-la-diabetes
- https://www.significados.com/ozonoterapia/
- https://definicion.de/acupuntura/
- https://www.botanical-online.com/medicina-natural/flores-bach-diabetes
- http://www.redgdps.org/guia-de-diabetes-tipo-2-para-clinicos/6-educacion-terapeutica-en-diabetes-20180917
- http://diabeweb.com/blog/18/apoyo-psicologico-diabetes
- http://diabetesdietas.com/cuando-asistir-grupo-apoyo-la-diabetes/

Topic II. Obesity

Chapter 1. Concept
- https://www.healthychildren.org/Spanish/health-issues/conditions/obesity/Paginas/body-mass-index-formula.aspxhttps://obymed.es/tipos-de-obesidad/

Chapter 2. Most frequent causes
- https://www.elconfidencial.com/alma-corazon-vida/2016-10-06/medicamentos-engordan_1270838/
- https://www.elsevier.es/es-revista-endocrinologia-nutricion-12-articulo-funcion-endocrina-obesidad-S1575092211002361
- https://www.mayoclinic.org/es-es/diseases-conditions/cushing-syndrome/symptoms-causes/syc-20351310
- https://www.sanitas.es/sanitas/seguros/es/particulares/biblioteca-de-salud/dieta-alimentacion/adelgazar-sobrepeso/hipotiroidismo-obesidad.html

- https://www.mayoclinic.org/es-es/diseases-conditions/male-hypogonadism/symptoms-causes/syc-20354881
- https://www.fesemi.org/informacion-pacientes/conozca-mejor-su-enfermedad/acromegalia-y-gigantismo
- https://www.intramed.net/contenidover.asp?contenidoid=94048
- http://obesidadinfantil.consumer.es/web/es/padres_obesos/1.php
- https://www.elsevier.es/es-revista-endocrinologia-nutricion-12-articulo-obesidad-adipogenesis-resistencia-insulina-S1575092211100218X
- https://laboratoriosniam.com/la-estrecha-relacion-entre-sop-y-obesidad/
- https://www.mayoclinic.org/es-es/diseases-conditions/male-hypogonadism/symptoms-causes/syc-20354881

Chapter 3. Most common symptoms

- https://cuidateplus.marca.com/enfermedades/ginecologicas/amenorrea.html
- https://kidshealth.org/es/teens/acanthosis-esp.html
- https://portal.hospitalclinic.org/enfermedades/obesidad/sintomas
- https://www.mayoclinic.org/es-es/diseases-conditions/stretch-marks/symptoms-causes/syc-20351139

Chapter 4. Associated diseases

- https://www.cmed.es/actualidad/la-obesidad-y-sus-enfermedades-asociadas_306.html
- https://vitaliv.app/esta-relacionado-el-exceso-de-colesterol-con-el-exceso-de-peso/
- cielo.isciii.es/scielo.php?script=sci_arttext&pid=S1137-66272004000300006
- https://funcionales.es/obesidad-dietas-ricas-en-grasa-y-alteraciones-de-la-motilidad-intestinal
- http://www.ilsoeducacion.com/150-litiasis-vesicular-y-obesidad
- http://www.scielo.org.pe/scielo.php?script=sci_arttext&pid=S1025-55832017000200016
- https://cuidateplus.marca.com/enfermedades/digestivas/colon-irritable.html

- https://cuidateplus.marca.com/enfermedades/urologicas/litiasis-renal.html
- https://www.revistanefrologia.com/es-obesidad-enfermedad-renal-consecuencias-ocultas-articulo-S0211699517300553

Chapter 5. Consequences
- https://medlineplus.gov/spanish/metabolicsyndrome.html
- https://www.sdpnoticias.com/estilo-de-vida/2015/11/22/hablemos-de-la-osteoartrosis-artrosis-o-enfermedad-articular-degenerativa
- https://mejorconsalud.com/6-consejos-para-eliminar-naturalmente-los-acrocordones/
- https://www.salud.mapfre.es/enfermedades/dermatologicas/que-son-y-como-tratar-los-acrocordones/
- ttps://www.mayoclinic.org/es-es/diseases-conditions/nonalcoholic-fatty-liver-disease/symptoms-causes/syc-20354567
- http://chemocare.com/es/chemotherapy/side-effects/Hiperuricemia.aspx
- https://www.webconsultas.com/salud-al-dia/esteatosis-hepatica/prevencion-de-la-esteatosis-hepatica
- https://www.mayoclinic.org/es-es/diseases-conditions/metabolic-syndrome/symptoms-causes/syc-20351916

Chapter 6. Treatments
- https://medlineplus.gov/spanish/ency/patientinstructions/000346.htm
- https://www.laparoscopic.md/es/questions/cirugia-bariatrica/cuales-son-los-posibles-efectos-secundarios-de-la-cirugia-bariatrica
- https://cuidateplus.marca.com/belleza-y-piel/diccionario/lipoescultura.html
- https://www.clinicasobesitas.com/obesidad/cirugia-plastica-obesidad/
- https://www.hmhospitales.com/usuario-hm/apuntes-de-salud/cirugia-de-la-obesidad-(bariatrica)
- https://www.mayoclinic.org/es-es/tests-procedures/bariatric-surgery/about/pac-20394258

Chapter 7. Physical activity
- www.bbc.com/mundo/noticias/2015/08/150807_salud_recomendaciones_ejercicio_personas_sobrepeso_ig

- https://www.clinicasobesitas.com/actualidad/ejercicio-fisico-adaptado-a-la-obesidad/
- https://pierdepesoencasa.com/ejercicios-para-obesos-morbidos-sedentarios-casa/

Chapter 8. Dietary measures
- https://www.elsevier.es/es-revista-offarm-4-articulo-dietas-hipocaloricas-13070732
- https://www.fundacionbengoa.org/informacion_nutricion/dietas-moda.asp
- https://www.mayoclinic.org/es-es/healthy-lifestyle/nutrition-and-healthy-eating/in-depth/glycemic-index-diet/art-20048478
- http://saludyalimentacion.consumer.es/obesidad/alimentos-aconsejados-permitidos-y-limitados
- https://encolombia.com/libreria-digital/lmedicina/obesidad-carta/obesicart-gc-capitulo14a/
- https://www.hogarmania.com/cocina/recetas/pescados-mariscos/201803/salmonetes-setas-tomates-39424.html

Chapter 9. Vitamins and Minerals
- https://myemail.constantcontact.com/LA-CARENCIA-DE-VITAMINAS-Y-MINERALES-INFLUYE-PARA-LA-OBESIDAD-EN-ADULTOS.html?soid=1116729122843&aid=eNYZOiXSYkc
- https://www.clinicabaviera.com/blog/mundo-bavieraconoce-que-alimentos-tienen-vitamina-a/
- https://www.eldiario.es/consumoclaro/comer/frutas-verduras-vitamina-C-naranjas_0_810869830.html
- https://www.crbard.com/vab-guide/El-Blog-de-BAV/VitaminaE-beneficios-y-alimentos
- https://www.hola.com/cocina/nutricion/200905228505/minerales/calcio/hierro/
- https://rpp.pe/lima/actualidad/fortalece-tus-huesos-con-alimentos-ricos-en-calcio-y-vitamina-d-noticia-633557

Chapter 10. Medicinal plants
- https://www.hogarmania.com/salud/salud-familiar/remedios-naturales/201610/plantas-medicinales-ayudan-quemar-grasa-33845.html

- https://mejorconsalud.com/11-mejores-plantas-para-bajar-de-peso/
- https://www.portalsalud.com/hierbas-para-la-resistencia-a-la-insulina_13125095/
- https://www.hogarmania.com/salud/salud-familiar/remedios-naturales/201610/plantas-medicinales-ayudan-quemar-grasa-33845.html
- https://www.salud180.com/salud-z/plantas-medicinales-contra-la-obesidad

Chapter 11. Natural supplements
- https://as.com/deporteyvida/2017/06/20/portada/1497954710_295576.html
- https://imeoobesidad.com/blog/suplementos-dieteticos-perder-peso/

Chapter 12. Alternative therapies
- https://www.salud180.com/salud-dia-a-dia/5-terapias-para-controlar-el-estres
- https://www.lanacion.com.ar/ciencia/dos-terapias-permiten-corregir-una-imagen-corporal-distorsionada-nid1252757
- https://cuidateplus.marca.com/enfermedades/psiquiatricas/trastorno-por-atracon.html
- https://medlineplus.gov/spanish/ency/patientinstructions/000874.htm
- https://www.efe.com/efe/espana/gente/hedonismo-alimentario-el-placer-por-comer-productos-saludables/10007-2885261
- https://www.elsevier.com/es-es/connect/estudiantes-de-ciencias-de-la-salud/tecnicas-cognitivo-conductuales-para-afrontar-el-estres-de-los-examenes
- https://cuidateplus.marca.com/belleza-y-piel/diccionario/risoterapia.html
- https://cnnespanol.cnn.com/2017/10/17/8-claves-para-acabar-con-la-adiccion-a-los-carbohidratos/

Topic III. Thyroid Gland Diseases

Chapter 1. Concept
- https://medlineplus.gov/spanish/thyroiddiseases.html
- https://medlineplus.gov/spanish/hypothyroidism.html

- https://www.mayoclinic.org/es-es/diseases-conditions/hashimotos-disease/symptoms-causes/syc-20351855
- https://medlineplus.gov/spanish/hyperthyroidism.html
- https://medlineplus.gov/spanish/ency/article/001178.htm

Chapter 2. Most frequent causes
- https://www.cuidatutiroides.com/t/hipotiroidismo_hereditarios/
- https://www.mayoclinic.org/es-es/diseases-conditions/hyperthyroidism/symptoms-causes/syc-20373659

Chapter 3. Most common symptoms
- https://www.mayoclinic.org/es-es/diseases-conditions/hypothyroidism/symptoms-causes/syc-20350284
- https://cuidateplus.marca.com/enfermedades/digestivas/hipertiroidismo.html
- https://www.mayoclinic.org/es-es/diseases-conditions/hashimotos-disease/symptoms-causes/syc-20351855
- https://www.mayoclinic.org/es-es/diseases-conditions/goiter/symptoms-causes/syc-20351829

Chapter 4. Associated diseases
- https://www.navarrozarza.com.mx/?p=420
- https://www.sanitas.es/sanitas/seguros/es/particulares/biblioteca-de-salud/prevencion-salud/tiroides-depresion.html
- https://www.mayoclinic.org/es-es/diseases-conditions/secondary-hypertension/symptoms-causes/syc-20350679
- https://www.mayoclinic.org/es-es/diseases-conditions/hypothyroidism/expert-answers/hypothyroidism/faq-20057789
- https://espanol.mercola.com/boletin-de-salud/muchos-sintomas-que-sugieren-una-tiroides-lenta.aspx

Chapter 5. Consequences
- https://www.informajoven.org/info/salud/K_7_4.asp
- https://comerparavenceralcancer.com/2018/09/25/los-alimentos-basicos-para-vencer-al-cancer/

- https://www.cancer.org/es/cancer/cancer-de-tiroides/causas-riesgos-prevencion/prevencion.html
- https://www.elsevier.es/es-revista-revista-medica-clinica-las-condes-202-articulo-disfuncion-tiroidea-y-corazon-S0716864015000395
- https://www.cuerpomente.com/salud-natural/terapias-naturales/como-prevenir-tiroiditis_2181
- https://medlineplus.gov/spanish/ency/article/000683.htm
- https://mejorconsalud.com/bebidas-tratar-hipertiroidismo/
- https://www.tuasaude.com/es/remedios-caseros-para-el-hipotiroidismo/
- https://www.evafertilityclinics.es/novedades-inseminacion-artificial/tiroides-y-fertilidad-femenina/

Chapter 6. Treatments
- https://www.hormone.org/pacientes-y-cuidadores/medicines-for-hypothyroidism
- https://www.cancer.org/es/cancer/cancer-de-tiroides/despues-del-tratamiento/cuidado-de-seguimiento.html
- https://medlineplus.gov/spanish/ency/article/002933.htm
- https://www.radiologyinfo.org/sp/info.cfm?pg=radioiodine
- https://www.cun.es/enfermedades-tratamientos/cuidados-casa/cuidados-tras-yodo-radiactivo
- https://www.barnaclinic.com/blog/cirugia-de-tiroides/cuidados-en-casa-cirugia-de-tiroides/
- https://www.cancer.org/es/cancer/cancer-de-tiroides/tratamiento/yodo-radioactivo.html
- https://www.barnaclinic.com/blog/cirugia-de-tiroides/complicaciones-frecuentes-cirugia-de-tiroides/
- https://medlineplus.gov/spanish/druginfo/meds/a682461-es.html

Chapter 7. Physical activity
- http://scielo.sld.cu/scielo.php?script=sci_arttext&pid=S0864-03002017000300013
- https://www.portalsalud.com/ejercicio-afecta-produccion-info_7609/
- https://www.barnaclinic.com/blog/cirugia-de-tiroides/recuperacion-cirugia-tiroides-reposo/

Chapter 8. Dietary measures

- https://www.tuasaude.com/es/dieta-para-la-intolerancia-a-la-lactosa/
- https://www.aecat.net/consejos-practicos/terapiacon-yodo-radioactivo/dieta-baja-en-yodo-y-otras-recomendaciones/
- https://www.mayoclinic.org/es-es/diseases-conditions/lactose-intolerance/symptoms-causes/syc-20374232
- https://www.cuerpomente.com/alimentacion/dieta-terapeutica/recetas-equilibrar-tiroides-hormonas_1778
- https://belleza.trendencias.com/?utm_source=bebesymas&utm_medium=network&utm_campaign=favicons
- http://www.contigosalud.com/menu-para-hipotiroidismo
- https://positive.varilux.es/bienestar/intolerancia-gluten/
- https://shawellnessclinic.com/es/shamagazine/recomendaciones-nutricionales-para-hipotiroidismo-e-hipertiroidismo/

Chapter 9. Vitamins and minerals

- https://www.infobae.com/salud/2018/05/25/hipo-e-hipertiroidismo-cuales-son-los-seis-nutrientes-esenciales-para-su-buen-funcionamiento/
- https://www.alimente.elconfidencial.com/bienestar/2019-04-15/selenio-mineral-gran-poder-antioxidante_1867706/

Chapter 10. Medicinal plants

- https://www.promofarma.com/blog/salud-y-bienestar/4-plantas-para-aumentar-tus-defensas/
- https://www.revistaciencias.unam.mx/es/160-revistas/revista-ciencias-15/1411-%C2%BFplantas-que-producen-cancer.html
- https://es.wikipedia.org/wiki/Sustancias_t%C3%B3xicas_vegetales
- https://rolloid.net/7-hierbas-naturales-tratar-los-problemas-tiroides/
- http://www.consumer.es/web/es/alimentacion/aprender_a_comer_bien/enfermedad/2010/01/29/190795.php

Chapter 11. Natural supplements

- https://laopinion.com/guia-de-compras/los-mejores-10-suplementos-para-el-cuidado-de-la-tiroides/

Chapter 12. Alternative therapies

- https://www.telesurtv.net/news/8-alternativas-para-disminuir-el-estres--20150922-0010.html

- https://www.telesurtv.net/news/8-alternativas-para-disminuir-el-estres--20150922-0010.html
- https://www.cuerpomente.com/blogs/come-limpio/ayuno-tipos-contraindicaciones_2542
- https://gabinetedepsicologia.com/tratamiento-de-la-tristeza-psicologos-madrid-tres-cantos

Topic IV. Polycystic Ovary Syndrome

Chapter 1. Concept
- https://medlineplus.gov/spanish/ency/article/000369.htm
- https://kidshealth.org/es/teens/pcos-esp.html

Chapter 2. Most frequent causes
- https://aesopspain.org/sop-y-hipotiroidismo/
- https://medlineplus.gov/spanish/ency/article/000348.htm
- https://www.msdmanuals.com/es/professional/trastornos-endocrinos-y-metab%C3%B3licos/trastornos-hipofisarios/gigantismo-y-acromegalia
- https://es.familydoctor.org/condicion/resistencia-la-insulina/
- https://kidshealth.org/es/teens/pcos-esp.html
- https://www.hormone.org/audiences/pacientes-y-cuidadores/preguntas-y-respuestas/2010/sindrome-de-ovario-poliquistico

Chapter 3. Most common symptoms
- https://kidshealth.org/es/teens/pcos-esp.html
- https://laboratoriosniam.com/la-estrecha-relacion-entre-sop-y-obesidad/
- https://www.infosalus.com/enfermedades/ginecologia/ovarios-poliquisticos/que-es-ovarios-poliquisticos-62.html

Chapter 4. Associated diseases
- http://www.scielo.br/scielo.php?pid=S0066-782X2010000500010&script=sci_arttext&tlng=es
- https://www.elsevier.es/es-revista-revista-medica-clinica-las-condes-202-articulo-sindrome-de-ovario-poliquistico-en-S0716864016300633

- https://www.crbard.com/vab-guide/Saber-mas/Palpacion-de-los-cambios-fibroquisticos-de-la-mama

Chapter 5. Long term consequences
- https://www.infosalus.com/asistencia/noticia-mujeres-sindrome-ovario-poliquistico-tienen-mayor-riesgo-sufrir-enfermedades-cardiovasculares-20100519142806.html
- http://cardiosalus.com/salud/reportajes/como-se-puede-prevenir-la-cardiopatia-isquemica.html
- https://www.cuerpomente.com/blogs/come-limpio/sindrome-ovarios-poliquisticos_1638
- https://www.organicfacts.net/remedios-caseros/sindrome-de-ovario-poliquistico.html?lang=es
- https://mejorconsalud.com/tratamiento-natural-para-el-sindrome-de-los-ovarios-poliquisticos/
- https://www.infosalus.com/salud-investigacion/noticia-mujeres-sindrome-ovario-poliquistico-tienen-doble-riesgo-ser-ingresadas-otros-trastornos-20150128094134.html

Chapter 6. Treatments
- https://espanol.womenshealth.gov/a-z-topics/polycystic-ovary-syndrome
- https://medlineplus.gov/spanish/druginfo/meds/a699055-es.html
- https://www.breastcancer.org/es/tratamiento/cirugia/preventiva_ovarios/preventiva_ovarios/durante
- https://medlineplus.gov/spanish/assistedreproductivetechnology.html
- https://www.breastcancer.org/es/tratamiento/cirugia/preventiva_ovarios/riesgos

Chapter 7. Physical activity
- https://www.fisiologiadelejercicio.com/sindrome-de-ovario-poliquistico-y-entrenamiento-fisico/
- https://www.adamedmujer.com/trastornos/ejercicio-fisico-para-mujeres-con-sindrome-de-ovarios-poliquisticos/

Chapter 8. Dietary measures
- https://youngwomenshealth.org/2006/05/15/nutricion-para-sopq/
- https://www.directoalpaladar.com/ingredientes-y-alimentos/las-mejores-recetas-con-nueces-de-directo-al-paladar

- https://laboratoriosniam.com/si-tienes-sop-estos-deliciosos-alimentos-seran-tus-mejores-amigos/
- https://www.elespanol.com/cocinillas/recetas/verduras/20150422/brocoli-gratinado-jamon-queso-huevo-receta-facil/1000111038898_30.html
- https://informalia.eleconomista.es/informalia/belleza/noticias/8578741/08/17/Toma-nota-estos-son-los-alimentos-para-combatir-el-acne-.html
- http://www.diabetes.org/es/alimentos-y-actividad-fisica/alimentos/que-voy-a-comer/comprension-de-los-carbohidratos/indice-glucemico-y-diabetes.html
- https://laboratoriosniam.com/si-tienes-sop-reduce-tus-niveles-de-testosterona-con-estos-5-alimentos/
- http://muysaludable.sanitas.es/nutricion/dietas-hipocaloricas-consisten/
- http://muysaludable.sanitas.es/nutricion/dietas-hipocaloricas-consisten/

Chapter 9. Vitamins and minerals
- https://www.facebook.com/AdiosQuistesDeOvario/photos/7-vitaminas-y-minerales-para-eliminar-el-sindrome-de-ovario-poliquisticovitamina/812927655559095/
- https://www.hsnstore.com/blog/colina-e-inositol/
- https://www.sabervivirtv.com/nutricion/alimentos-ricos-en-zinc-beneficios_1990/5
- https://www.zonadiet.com/nutricion/cromo.htm
- https://ods.od.nih.gov/factsheets/VitaminD-DatosEnEspanol/
- https://medlineplus.gov/spanish/ency/article/002404.htm
- https://www.oftalvist.es/blog/alimentos-ricos-vitamina-a-para-la-vista/

Chapter 10. Medicinal plants
- https://laboratoriosniam.com/si-tienes-sop-reduce-tus-niveles-de-testosterona-con-estos-5-alimentos/
- https://www.mujerhoy.com/vivir/madres/201810/08/plantas-aumentan-fertilidad-601178454434-ga.html

- https://culturacolectiva.com/estilo-de-vida/como-bajar-los-niveles-de-testosterona-si-eres-mujer
- https://www.montevideo.com.uy/Mujer/Plantas-medicinales-para-regularizar-la-menstruacion-uc322492
- https://www.enbuenasmanos.com/tratamientos-para-la-resistencia-a-la-insulina

Chapter 11. Natural supplements
- https://www.amazon.es/NIAM-S-Ovario-Poliqu%C3%ADstico-C%C3%A1psulas/dp/B01EHSNIW2/ref=pd_lpo_sbs_121_t_0/260-3033207-7492715?_encoding=UTF8&psc=1&refRID=M6DQXEH1DAE2SR16TDYY
- https://www.guiadesuplementos.es/melatonina/
- https://miriamginecologia.com/blog/sindrome-de-ovarios-poliquisticos-parte-iv/
- https://www.guiadesuplementos.es/acido-folico/

Chapter 12. Alternative therapies
- https://www.eluniversal.com.co/blogs/entendiendo-la-piel-con-wilmar-polo/terapias-alternativas-y-complementarias-en-tratamientos-cutaneos
- https://www.todopapas.com/fertilidad/fertilidad-en-la-mujer/fertilidad-acupuntura-y-otras-terapias-alternativas-5615
- https://www.vix.com/es/imj/salud/5334/las-mejores-terapias-alternativas-para-bajar-de-peso
- https://mejorconsalud.com/tratamiento-natural-para-el-exceso-de-vello/
- https://es.wikipedia.org/wiki/Fitoterapia
- https://www.hedonai.com/tratamientos-faciales/acne/
- https://www.hablandodehomeopatia.com/como-tratar-el-acne-con-medicamentos-homeopaticos/

Topic V. Menopause and Andropause

Chapter 1. Concept
- https://definicion.de/climaterio/

- https://cuidateplus.marca.com/sexualidad/diccionario/menopausia.html
- http://www.scielo.org.bo/scielo.php?script=sci_arttext&pid=S1012-29662006000200011
- https://www.msdmanuals.com/es/hogar/salud-femenina/trastornos-menstruales-y-sangrados-vaginales-an%C3%B3malos/menopausia-prematura
- https://www.clinicalascondes.cl/BLOG/Listado/Ginecologia/Climaterio-y-Menopausia

Chapter 2. Most frequent causes
- https://espanol.womenshealth.gov/menopause/early-or-premature-menopause

Chapter 3. Most common symptoms
- https://www.salud.mapfre.es/salud-familiar/hombre/recomendaciones/menopausia-masculina/
- http://www.davila.cl/menopausia-y-climaterio-sintomas-y-tratamiento/

Chapter 4. Associated diseases
- http://scielo.isciii.es/scielo.php?script=sci_arttext&pid=S0212-16112006000900001
- https://www.mayoclinic.org/es-es/diseases-conditions/high-blood-pressure/expert-answers/menopause-and-high-blood-pressure/faq-20058406
- https://www.sabervivir.es/familia-saludable/mujer/vigila-mas-tu-tiroides-en-la-menopausia
- https://www.msdmanuals.com/es/hogar/trastornos-hormonales-y-metab%C3%B3licos/trastornos-relacionados-con-el-colesterol/dislipidemia-dislipemia
- https://www.drfcarmona.com/menopausia/enfermedades-asociadas-la-menopausia/

Chapter 5. Consequences
- https://fundaciondelcorazon.com/ejercicio/ejercicio-fisico/3175-cardiopatia-isquemica.html
- https://www.cuerpomente.com/salud-natural/consultorio/regenerar-masa-osea-osteoporosis-forma-natural_2792

- https://mifarmaciaespana.com/tratamientos-naturales-para-la-disfuncion-erectil-una-solucion-efectiva-y-saludable/

Chapter 6. Treatments
- https://www.vademecum.es/enfermedad-menopausia+(climaterio+femenino)_424_3
- https://www.clinicalascondes.cl/NOTICIAS/Andropausia,-el-bajon-hormonal-de-los-hombres
- https://cuidateplus.marca.com/belleza-y-piel/medicina-estetica/2018/11/16/consecuencias-implantes-pelo-realizados-turquia-168131.html
- https://www.20minutos.es/noticia/565418/0/cirugia/vaginal/riesgos/
- https://espanol.womenshealth.gov/menopause/menopause-treatment
- ttps://www.todopapas.com/medicamentos/hormonas/progyluton
- https://www.webconsultas.com/belleza-y-bienestar/tratamientos-esteticos/que-es-la-c
- https://vilarovira.com/cirugia-genital-masculina/
- https://medlineplus.gov/spanish/druginfo/meds/a601041-es.html
- https://www.diariofemenino.com/articulos/salud/menopausia/cirugia-estetica-durante-la-etapa-de-la-menopausia/

Chapter 7. Physical activity
- https://www.webconsultas.com/ejercicio-y-deporte/ejercicio-en-las-etapas-de-la-vida/ejercicios-apropiados-en-la-menopausia-1937
- https://www.webconsultas.com/ejercicio-y-deporte/ejercicio-en-las-etapas-de-la-vida/ejercicio-en-la-menopausia-1935
- https://www.webconsultas.com/ejercicio-y-deporte/ejercicio-en-las-etapas-de-la-vida/beneficios-del-ejercicio-en-la-menopausia-193

Chapter 8. Dietary measures
- https://cuidateplus.marca.com/sexualidad/diccionario/afrodisiacos.html
- https://www.dietacoherente.com/recetas-para-la-menopausia-ensaladas-potajes/
- https://sevilla.abc.es/gurme/las-mejores-recetas/10-recetas-con-calabacin/

- https://holadoctor.com/es/%C3%A1lbum-de-fotos/el-mejor-men%C3%BA-durante-la-menopausia-ayuda-a-evitar-la-suba-de-peso-y-el-estr%C3%A9s
- https://contenidos.bupasalud.com/salud-bienestar/vida-bupa/alimentaci%C3%B3n-saludable
- https://www.miqueridamenopausia.com/que-son-las-fitohormonas/
- https://www.huercasa.com/es/blog/alimentos-antioxidantes
- https://www.directoalpaladar.com/salud/como-aprovechar-mejor-los-nutrientes-en-la-cocina
- https://mifarmaciaespana.com/conoce-los-afrodisiacos-naturales-mas-efectivos-y-disfruta-de-tu-sexualidad/

Chapter 9. Vitamins and minerals
- https://www.hola.com/estar-bien/20180831128919/vitaminas-y-minerales-en-la-menopausia-cs/
- https://www.miarevista.es/salud/fotos/7-alimentos-con-un-plus-de-vitamina-c/vitamina-c-1
- https://www.danone.es/es/salud/tendencias/alimentos-calcio-no-lacteos.html
- https://www.globalhealingcenter.net/salud-natural/alimentos-vitamina-c.html
- https://medlineplus.gov/spanish/ency/article/002406.htm
- https://laopinion.com/guia-de-compras/3-vitaminas-y-minerales-que-necesitas-consumir-durante-la-menopausia-para-fortalecer-tu-salud/

Chapter 10. Medicinal plants
- https://articulos.mercola.com/sitios/articulos/archivo/2014/11/08/hierbas-y-especias-para-bajar-de-peso.aspx
- https://www.eldinamo.cl/ambiente/2016/05/09/plantas-hierbas-combatir-estres-depresion/
- https://www.autocrecimiento.com/salud/plantas-medicinales-trastornos-menstruales/
- https://www.cuerpomente.com/salud-natural/tratamientos/sofocos-remedios-naturales_2133
- https://holadoctor.com/es/%C3%A1lbum-de-fotos/los-10-mejores-t%C3%A9s-para-dormir-bien
- https://mejorconsalud.com/hierbas-medicinales-que-nos-aportan-energia/

- https://www.promofarma.com/blog/salud-y-bienestar/descubre-las-5-plantas-que-equilibran-tus-hormonas/

Chapter 11. Natural supplements
- https://www.hsnstore.com/blog/menopausia-suplementos-naturales/

Chapter 12. Alternative therapies
- https://www.subz3ro.mx/7-terapias-alternativas-disminuir-estres/
- https://www.mindalia.com/noticias/terapias-alternativas-bienestar-salud-naturales/
- https://neurorhb.com/blog-dano-cerebral/que-es-la-terapia-ocupacional/
- https://www.diariofemenino.com/articulos/psicologia/ansiedad/terapias-alternativas-para-combatir-la-ansiedad/
- http://www.f-ima.org/es/factores-de-proteccion-para-la-prevencion/imagen-corporal
- https://articulos.mercola.com/sitios/articulos/archivo/2017/11/16/tratamientos-alternativos-para-la-depresion.aspx
- https://psicologiaymente.com/vida/tecnicas-relajacion-combatir-estres
- https://psicologiaymente.com/clinica/tecnicas-cognitivo-conductuales

The author

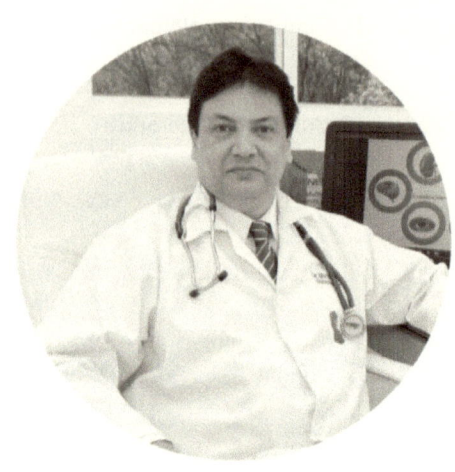

Dr. Mario Vega Carbó
Endocrinologist

* Cuban Physician graduated in 1994.
* Specialist in Endocrinology and Family Medicine.
* Master in Longevity and Ultrasonography.
* Professor of Medical Pathophysiology.
* Loving of doing what is good, family and nature.

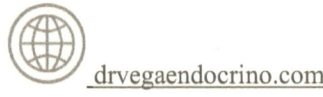 drvegaendocrino.com 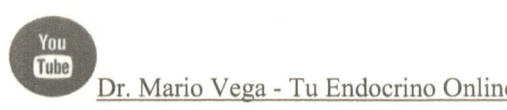 Dr. Mario Vega - Tu Endocrino Online

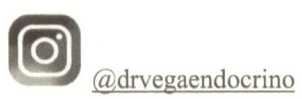 @drvegaendocrino 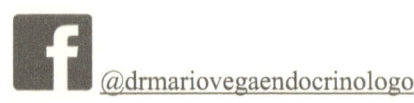 @drmariovegaendocrinologo

www.ingramcontent.com/pod-product-compliance
Lightning Source LLC
Chambersburg PA
CBHW030622220526
45463CB00004B/1380